Introduction

The year is 1700. It's almost dawn. At latest count, another 25 sailors aboard His Majesty's ship have taken ill. The journey has been long and treacherous. Many months have passed since the crew of hale and hearty men set sail across the high seas. Now, as the captain looks around him, his men are slowly dying, one by one. Their weakened, frail bodies are covered by mysterious, irregular patches of red and purple skin, their gums are swollen and bleeding, and many have lost their teeth. The scene just described was all too common among the sailing ships of the time. As a matter of fact, the condition had been known since the time of Hippocrates (400 B.C.). Yet, it wasn't until 1747 that a British doctor, James Lind, began to unravel the mystery behind this elusive killer by recognizing that men who were at sea for extended periods of time were being deprived of certain foods, particularly fresh fruits. And it wasn't until 1795 that the situation was remedied when the British issued supplies of lime juice to the sailors aboard their naval vessels. By what seemed to be a miracle, the elusive killer disappeared.

Why? What had this doctor discovered? What possible role could lime juice play in warding off this deadly ill that had plagued mankind for centuries?

Introduction

Since those days, it has been learned that the men on those long ocean voyages were suffering the effects of vitamin C deficiency. And the dreaded killer was a condition known to us today as scurvy.

Throughout most of history no one knew about the existence of vitamins or minerals. Well, not by name, anyway. People only knew the *results* of either having or not having them in their diet.

The human diet would undergo changes according to the food supplies that were readily available. At times, the diet would be sufficiently balanced to keep a population healthy and thriving. At other times, the diet would be deficient in various essential nutrients, and a population would suffer the consequences. Sometimes when this would occur, people tried to change their diet, recognizing in some elementary way the connection between good food and good health. In this sense, then, even without the knowledge that we have now, people did make attempts to deal with vitamin and mineral deficiencies and determine what foods contribute to a healthy life.

Today, of course, we have a wealth of knowledge about these nutrients. In fact, we are so bombarded with vitamin and mineral advertisements, books, newspaper articles, and magazine stories that it's almost difficult to imagine how people existed without all this information. Not only do we have facts about what each of these nutrients will do for us when we consume them in normal amounts, but we now have hoards of claims about what effects they may have if we take them in extremely large doses. For example, one report says a megadose of vitamin A can cure cancer, while another says the same nutrient can be toxic and is dangerous for pregnant women. Now we have a new problem . . . which report do we believe?

Some of the claims promote ideas that seem really tempting. Take a little of this vitamin, they'll say, or a large dose of that mineral, and you'll be able to grow hair, smooth wrinkles, avoid cancer, and stop the aging process. Who couldn't be seduced by such fantastic promises?

But stop and think—if it were really that easy, if all these claims were true, then no one would ever get cancer, go bald, wrinkle, or look a day over 25. We'd be an overwhelmingly healthy society that looked young forever! But, as we all know, this just isn't the case. The inconsistency is founded in the fact that most of what is reported about vitamins and minerals is anecdotal information—hearsay—the "it worked for me, so you try it" type of advice. Following advice based on this kind of claim may actually endanger your health and will most certainly waste your money. The kind of advice you can use and trust should be based *not on hearsay,* but rather *on scientific evidence*—evidence that's supported by repeated studies, tests, and long, hard hours of research. So, where do you find this kind of advice?

Right here. To help you sort through the confusing array of information that's available, CONSUMER GUIDE® and a team of recognized experts in the

Introduction

field of nutrition have provided you with a thorough, medically sound, up-to-date sourcebook. We've cut through the confusion and come up with a clear explanation of each nutrient's function, value, and dangers of deficiency and overdose.

In the *Complete Book of Vitamins and Minerals* you can find answers to such questions as: Which ones do I need? How much of each should I take? What foods are rich sources? What about supplements? Are there any benefits in taking large doses to help prevent or cure a disease? Are there any dangers? What's the latest research?

To present the material in this book in the most straightforward way possible, we're going to deal with it in the following way. First, we'll explain how the challenge of eating right is *really up to you*. Then, to help you understand something about what good nutrition provides, we'll tell you everything you *need* to know about vitamins and minerals. Finally, should your doctor determine that you need supplements, we'll tell you everything you may *want* to know about those that are most popularly prescribed. Since we emphasize that eating a balanced diet with the recommended nutrient intakes is your best nutrition insurance, it's our hope that the information in the book compels you to consciously select food that will contribute to a healthier life.

Well then. What are you waiting for? You have a lot of healthy living—*and* eating—to do. So read on and enjoy. And, oh yes, one more thing . . . here's to your good health!

Chapter 1

Eating Right Is Up to You

Studying only vitamins or minerals in the school of nutrition is like studying only verbs or nouns in an English class. It's also necessary to understand what food contains, why we need it, and how it's used in our bodies. Only then can we understand the intricate workings of foods' essential nutrients. With this knowledge, we have it within our power to eat better and live a healthier life.

Nutrition can be defined as the sum of the processes by which an animal or plant absorbs and uses food substances. To understand what nutrition and eating right really mean, it's necessary to know something about the composition of food and about metabolism. And, of course, it's also important to recognize the nutritive values in the foods you eat.

History

People have walked the face of the earth for at least 250,000 years. For most of that time they were hunt-

Eating Right Is Up to You

ers and gatherers, scrounging for food among the plants and animals. When food sources became scarce, tribes and individuals moved on to greener pastures . . . or perished.

About 10,000 years ago, human beings developed agriculture. They began to farm and to domesticate animals, thereby working with the environment to take care of themselves. From ignorance evolved curiosity about how food sustains life. With the dawning of the scientific age, people began to ask questions. What happens to food when it is eaten? How does food generate energy? What foods are important for growth and the maintenance of life? These and other questions could not be answered until chemistry, biochemistry, physiology, and other related sciences had advanced.

In the late 1700s, Antoine Lavoisier, a Frenchman often considered the "Father of Nutrition," investigated the relationship between respiration and energy production. His studies showed that our bodies use the oxygen in the air we inhale to produce body heat and energy. He also observed that, in the process, carbon dioxide is created and exhaled. Lavoisier concluded that the food we eat acts as fuel, which is oxidized or "burned up" in the body to release energy. This body process has been compared to a "slow furnace." In a coal furnace, for example, coal burns in the presence of oxygen and releases carbon dioxide and energy in the form of heat. In a sense, the oxidation of food is a similar process. In the presence of oxygen, the food we take in is "burned" to release carbon dioxide and energy.

Eating Right Is Up to You

Lavoisier's work was the first step to uncovering how food is used to sustain life. But the oxidation of food is only a part of a complex series of reactions that occur within the body—reactions that are cumulatively referred to as *metabolism.*

Metabolism and Energy

Metabolism applies to all the chemical reactions that take place within each of the body's billions of cells. Every minute of every day our cells are busy breaking down the molecules of certain substances and building up the molecules of others. These chemical reactions are necessary for the production of hundreds of compounds that are vital for life. The proteins of muscles, the hormones, the enzymes, the fats, and the stored forms of sugar are examples of such necessary compounds. As a result of these complex reactions, chemical waste products are produced as well and must be eliminated from the body. And, of course, all-important energy is either stored or released as these reactions are taking place.

What is energy? Energy is simply the *ability to do work.* Today, we talk about the energy value of foods and about the number of calories that a particular food provides. The *calorie* is a unit of heat energy; that is, it measures energy as a form of heat. The energy value of individual foods depends on the amount of carbohydrates, fats, and proteins present. Measured in calories per gram, carbohydrates and proteins supply four calories per gram, and fats yield nine calories per gram. One gram is often described as equal to the mass of a paper clip. And here comes a mini-math lesson: There are 28.3 grams in an ounce and 453 grams in a pound. A milligram (mg) is $1/1,000$ of a gram; a microgram (μg) is $1/1,000,000$ of a gram, or $1/1,000$ of a milligram.

Different types of energy are interchangeable. For example, the chemical energy of carbohydrates, which are important body fuels, can be converted into heat energy to help maintain a constant body temperature. It can also be changed to kinetic energy necessary for muscle action and physical activity, or it can be trapped as chemical energy in other body compounds.

The Essential Nutrients

As the science of chemistry developed in the 18th and 19th centuries, so did procedures to analyze what we eat. Scientists soon discovered the great variety of chemically distinct compounds in foods. Ongoing experiments determined which foods and which parts of foods are best suited for growth and health.

In 1827, the English physician William Prout described the three "staminal principles" of foods necessary to support life: the oily, the saccharin, and the albuminous principles. These are recognized today as fats (and oils), carbohydrates, and proteins. Believing that a diet which supplies these substances would be nutritionally satisfactory, Prout was probably among the first to define an "adequate diet."

Eating Right Is Up to You

The study of food chemistry became increasingly sophisticated. Researchers began to use animals in their investigations. By the latter part of the 19th century, the "adequate diet" proposed by Prout was expanded to include inorganic elements, known as *minerals.* Today, at least sixteen minerals are recognized as essential nutrients for man.

By the dawning of the 20th century, a fifth class of nutrients was discovered. Scientists found that experimental animals perished if they were fed diets containing only highly purified preparations of fats, carbohydrates, proteins, and the known minerals. The missing vital nutrients turned out to be *vitamins.* (Previous researchers had failed to recognize the existence of vitamins because the diets prepared for experimental animals were not sufficiently "pure"; they were "contaminated" with vitamins.) Thirteen necessary vitamins are now known. The last, vitamin B_{12}, was discovered in the 1940s. Since these discoveries, the phrase "adequate diet" has been updated to refer to one that supplies all of these essential nutrients in appropriate amounts.

The table on pages 20-21 briefly describes the nature and function of the five classes of essential nutrients.

Recommended Dietary Allowances

The Recommended Daily Dietary Allowances, commonly referred to as the Recommended Dietary Allowances (RDAs), are established by the Food and Nutrition Board of the National Academy of Sciences,

Eating Right Is Up to You

National Research Council. The RDAs are estimates, based on available scientific knowledge, of the amount of nutrients that people need to maintain good health over a period of time. The RDAs are not intended to be used to evaluate an individual's food intake, though they are often used for that. The first RDA table was published in 1943, an outgrowth of the need to determine the food and nutrition situation in the United States as it related to national defense during World War II. The productivity of the American people depended upon good health, and good health depended upon good nutrition.

The first RDA list contained the recommended daily intake for calories, protein, six vitamins, and two minerals. To encompass new findings in the nutrition field, the RDAs have been revised periodically. We are currently using the 1980, 9th Revision, which consists of three tables. Table I, the main table (pages 22-25), gives "Recommended Daily Dietary Allowances" for protein, 10 vitamins, and six minerals divided into 17 different age/sex categories. Table II (pages 26-27) gives "Estimated Safe and Adequate Daily Dietary Intakes of Additional Selected Vitamins and Minerals." Less information is available about the 12 vitamins and minerals present in this table, and, therefore, more definite allowances can't be recommended. Table III (pages 28-29) provides "Mean Height and Weights and Recommended Energy Intakes" for 19 different age/sex categories.

RDAs are not minimum dietary requirements. They represent the amounts of nutrients that will meet the needs of normal, healthy people. With the exception of allowances for calories, the RDAs contain a "margin of safety." They are deliberately set at levels higher than estimated for the average person. This margin of safety allows for individual requirements and for those occasional but inevitable stress situations that occur in everyday life. This means you don't necessarily have to take in all of the quantities listed for each nutrient every day to be well nourished. Many authorities feel ⅔ or more of the RDA is adequate for most healthy people. However, RDAs are not intended to and cannot serve as guidelines for the nutritional management of seriously ill persons or of those with genetic or metabolic disorders that cause profound changes in nutrient needs.

The RDAs have been criticized because they have changed over the last 40 years and because they differ from the nutrient standards of other countries and those of international health organizations. These changes reflect growth as the RDAs are revised to incorporate new scientific data as it emerges. It is anticipated that the RDAs will be updated again in the near future.

The 1980, 9th Revision of the Recommended Daily Dietary Allowances are reproduced at the end of this chapter. The individual vitamin and mineral chapters which follow indicate the RDAs for men and women aged 23 to 50 where they have been established. You may refer back to the complete tables at the end of this chapter for information about the RDAs for infants, children, teenagers, and women who are pregnant or breast-feeding.

Eating Right Is Up to You

The "Basic Four" Food Groups

To help people plan and evaluate their diets for adequate nutrition, the United States Department of Agriculture developed the "Daily Food Guide." Commonly referred to as the "Basic Four" or the "Four Food Group Guide," this plan categorizes foods by their major nutrient contributions. Foods in the meat group—which includes nuts and dried beans and peas—are high in protein, for example, whereas fruits and vegetables are a good source of many vitamins, some of which are present only in small amounts in meats. Milk and milk products are excellent sources of calcium, an essential nutrient not provided in any significant amount by meats or cereals.

Daily diets that include the recommended number of servings from each of the four food groups will supply adequate amounts of the essential nutrients (with the possible exception of iron). The total amount of calories necessary depends upon an individual's age, sex, physical activity, and general health.

Teenage girls and women in their childbearing years may have trouble meeting the RDA for iron with usual diets because they need a relatively large amount of this trace element to replace what is lost during menstruation. Iron-rich foods, such as liver and foods fortified with iron, should be eaten frequently. Physicians and nutritionists often recommend iron supplements for girls and women to ensure an adequate intake.

Eating Right Is Up to You

A diet with only the minimum number of servings suggested by the Four Food Group plan furnishes about 1,200 calories—a good diet goal for people trying to lose weight. Physically active people and young people who are still growing need more than 1,200 calories. They should add more foods to the core diet to get those extra calories or foods included in the "Others" group. The "Others" group includes fats and oils (butter, margarine, salad dressings), sweets (sugar, candy, rich desserts), and beverages (soft drinks, alcoholic drinks). These are not included in any of the basic four groups because they have what nutritionists call a "low nutrient density" (popularly referred to as "empty calories"). They supply calories, but contribute little or no protein, vitamins, or minerals to the diet.

Not all the foods in any one of the four groups have the same nutritional value. For example, some foods in the fruit and vegetable group are much better sources of vitamin C or vitamin A than others. So the selections made to meet the daily recommendations for each group will affect the overall nutrient content of the diet.

The Four Food Group plan is not without its critics. Some argue that among the thousands of foods available there are many that do not fit well into any single group. Where does pizza belong, for example? With its sausage, cheese, tomato sauce, and crust, all four food groups are represented.

Dietary recommendations based on serving size may also be confusing. Certainly the quantity is not the same for all people. Although a serving of meat is usually considered as three ounces, this portion may be too much for some, too little for others.

Even though a diet may fulfill the recommendations of the Daily Food Guide, there is no guarantee that the RDAs for all nutrients will be achieved. Variety is the key. This may seem like an overly simplistic approach. But simplicity may make it easier to remember. And if it's easier to remember, we're more likely to do it. As we said, foods of similar nutritional value are grouped together in the Basic Four and each group has its own unique contribution to make. By varying the choices from each group from day to day, you will be assured of taking in a wide variety of needed nutrients. The Basic Four Plan *is* a useful guide to good nutrition.

Product Labeling

In response to the growing consumer interest in food values, the Food and Drug Administration (FDA) of the federal government instituted a means by which all consumer food goods can be labeled. The "Nutrition Information" panels on canned, frozen, and other packaged foods help consumers become familiar with nutrient terminology and guide them toward an intake of adequate amounts of the established essential nutrients.

More than half of all the food products regulated by the Food and Drug Administration carry nutrition labeling. Labeling is voluntary unless the manufacturer adds a nutrient to a food or makes a nutrition claim on the label. For example, a brand of cranberry juice fortified with vitamin C or a jar of peanut butter labeled "cholesterol free" would be required to have a nutrition label.

Since 1975, when nutrition labeling as we know it began, a nutrition label must provide percentages of the United States Recommended Daily Allowances (U.S. RDAs) for protein, vitamin A, vitamin C, thiamin, riboflavin, niacin, calcium, and iron. (Including information about seven additional vitamins and five minerals is optional.) The U.S. RDA is actually a simplification of the Recommended Dietary Allowances that were discussed earlier and represent a more complex set of nutrient needs based on age, sex, and body size. The extrapolated figures currently being used for the U.S. RDA are based on the 1968, 8th Revision of the RDA. The U.S. RDA for most nutrients is the highest RDA for all sex and age categories, excluding pregnant and lactating (nursing) women.

A typical nutrition label panel is shown on page 32. The number of servings in the package or container and the size of a single serving are shown on top. Next comes the amount of calories, protein, carbohydrates, and fat in one serving. This top section of the label may also provide information on the amount of cholesterol and sodium in a serving.

The second half of the nutrition label lists the percentages in the food of the U.S. RDA for protein and the five vitamins and two minerals mentioned earlier. In the sample label shown, one serving (one slice)

Eating Right Is Up to You

of wheat bread contains 8 percent of the U.S. RDA for thiamin, 6 percent for iron, and 0 percent for vitamin C. Using these figures and the U.S. RDA values given in the table on page 33, it is possible to calculate the actual amount of these nutrients as: 0.12 mg thiamin, 1.08 mg iron, and no vitamin C.

Even without going through the mathematics, you can use nutrition labeling to help you select food. A food that provides 10 percent of the U.S. RDA for a nutrient is considered a good source for that nutrient. Providing 50 percent or more would be an excellent source. Less than 10 percent shows that the food is an insignificant source of a nutrient. Nutrition labels can also be used to compare foods. For example, a comparison will show that canned peaches are a better source of vitamin A than canned pears.

Since 1984, the FDA has required the sodium content to be given on all foods that have a nutrition label. Foods labeled "sodium free" are those with less than 5 mg of sodium in a serving. "Very low sodium" foods must have 30 milligrams (mg) or less sodium in a serving. "Low sodium" foods are those with 140 mg or less in a serving. Manufacturers may also voluntarily list only the sodium content without a full nutrition label if nutrition labeling is not required on the food.

Nutrition labels help the dieter, too. A food high in nutrients but low in calories would be a wise choice. The FDA regulates many of the terms used on food labels. A food labeled "low calorie" may contain no more than 40 calories in a serving or 0.9 calories in a gram. A food labeled "reduced calorie" must have at least ⅓ less calories than the food it most closely resembles.

If you are a consumer who is sincerely interested in planning diets that are nutritionally sound, you have many tools to help you. The Basic Four is a simple, easy-to-use plan. Nutrition labeling provides more detailed information about the nutrient content of foods, and the RDA offers precise recommendations for most essential nutrients.

After reading this book, you should have a better understanding of the important contributions that vitamins and minerals make to good nutrition. And knowing that variety is the key to a healthy diet, planning your daily menus can be easy and fun. So remember, eating right really *is* up to you.

Eating Right Is Up to You

Classes of Essential Nutrients

Nutrient Class	Major Functions
Carbohydrates Starches; Sugars	Used primarily to supply energy; carbohydrates furnish 4 calories per gram.
Fats and Oils (Lipids) Essential fatty acids	Used to supply energy; fats furnish 9 calories per gram. A layer of fat under the skin insulates the body. Fat around internal organs cushions and protects them. Accumulation of too much fat leads to overweight and obesity. Dietary fat supplies the "essential fatty acids," important components of cells. The body cannot synthesize them.
Proteins Essential amino acids	Primary function is growth and maintenance of muscle or lean body tissues. Proteins can be used for energy, furnishing 4 calories per gram. Proteins are made up of smaller units—the amino acids—nine of which are essential; they cannot be made by the body.
Vitamins	Function as regulators of body chemistry or metabolism. Necessary for

Classes of Essential Nutrients (continued)

Nutrient Class	Major Functions
	normal synthesis and breakdown of body carbohydrates, fats, and proteins. Many play a role as coenzymes.
Inorganic Elements (Minerals)	As an important part of bones, some elements (e.g. calcium and phosphorus) contribute to body structure. Iron is a part of hemoglobin, the red pigment in blood that transports oxygen from the lungs to the tissues. Inorganic elements in body fluids help in maintaining acid-base balance and water balance. Some inorganic elements are essential for normal responses of nerves and muscles to stimuli. Certain inorganic elements are important regulators of body chemistry and are essential for normal enzyme action. Water accounts for 60 percent of body weight. Water is a constituent of every cell in the body. Blood, a water solution, carries nutrients to cells and waste products from them.

Table I*—Recommended Daily Dietary Allowances,[a] Revised 1980

Age (years)	Weight		Height	
	(kg)	(lbs)	(cm)	(in)
Infants				
0.0-0.5	6	13	60	24
0.5-1.0	9	20	71	28
Children				
1-3	13	29	90	35
4-6	20	44	112	44
7-10	28	62	132	52
Males				
11-14	45	99	157	62
15-18	66	145	176	69
19-22	70	154	177	70
23-50	70	154	178	70
51 +	70	154	178	70
Females				
11-14	46	101	157	62
15-18	55	120	163	64
19-22	55	120	163	64
23-50	55	120	163	64
51 +	55	120	163	64

Pregnancy
Lactating

* Designed for the maintenance of good nutrition of practically all healthy people in the U.S.A.

[a] The allowances are intended to provide for individual variations among most normal persons as they live in the United States under usual environmental stresses. Diets should be based on a variety of common foods in order to provide other nutrients for which human requirements have been less well defined. See pp. 28-29 for heights, weights and recommended intake.

Food and Nutrition Board, National Academy
of Sciences—National Research Council

Protein (g)	Fat-Soluble Vitamins		
	Vitamin A (μg R.E.)[b]	Vitamin D (μg)[c]	Vitamin E (mg α T.E.)[d]
kg × 2.2	420	10	3
kg × 2.0	400	10	4
23	400	10	5
30	500	10	6
34	700	10	7
45	1000	10	8
56	1000	10	10
56	1000	7.5	10
56	1000	5	10
56	1000	5	10
46	800	10	8
46	800	10	8
44	800	7.5	8
44	800	5	8
44	800	5	8
+30	+200	+5	+2
+20	+400	+5	+3

[b] Retinol equivalents. 1 Retinol equivalent = 1 μg retinol or 6 μg β carotene. See text for calculation of vitamin A activity of diets as retinol equivalents.

[c] As cholecalciferol. 10 μg cholecalciferol = 400 I.U. vitamin D.

[d] α-tocopheral equivalents. 1 mg d-α-tocopherol = 1 α T.E.

Table I (continued)—Recommended Daily Dietary Allowances,[a] Revised 1980

Age (years)	Water-Soluble Vitamins					
	Vitamin C (mg)	Thiamin (mg)	Ribo-flavin (mg)	Niacin (mg N.E.)[e]	Vitamin B6 (mg)	Folacin[f] (µg)
Infants						
0.0-0.5	35	0.3	0.4	6	0.3	30
0.5-1.0	35	0.5	0.6	8	0.6	45
Children						
1-3	45	0.7	0.8	9	0.9	100
4-6	45	0.9	1.0	11	1.3	200
7-10	45	1.2	1.4	16	1.6	300
Males						
11-14	50	1.4	1.6	18	1.8	400
15-18	60	1.4	1.7	18	2.0	400
19-22	60	1.5	1.7	19	2.2	400
23-50	60	1.4	1.6	18	2.2	400
51 +	60	1.2	1.4	16	2.2	400
Females						
11-14	50	1.1	1.3	15	1.8	400
15-18	60	1.1	1.3	14	2.0	400
19-22	60	1.1	1.3	14	2.0	400
23-50	60	1.0	1.2	13	2.0	400
51 +	60	1.0	1.2	13	2.0	400
Pregnancy	+20	+0.4	+0.3	+2	+0.6	+400
Lactating	+40	+0.5	+0.5	+5	+0.5	+100

[e] 1 N.E. (niacin equivalent) is equal to 1 mg of niacin or 60 mg of dietary tryptophan.

The folacin allowances refer to dietary sources as determined by *Lactobacillus casei* assay after treatment with enzymes ("conjugases") to make polyglutamyl forms of the vitamin available to the test organism.

Food and Nutrition Board, National Academy
of Sciences—National Research Council

Vitamin B12 (µg)	Minerals					
	Calcium (mg)	Phosphorus (mg)	Magnesium (mg)	Iron (mg)	Zinc (mg)	Iodine (µg)
0.5g	360	240	50	10	3	40
1.5	540	360	70	15	5	50
2.0	800	800	150	15	10	70
2.5	800	800	200	10	10	90
3.0	800	800	250	10	10	120
3.0	1200	1200	350	18	15	150
3.0	1200	1200	400	18	15	150
3.0	800	800	350	10	15	150
3.0	800	800	350	10	15	150
3.0	800	800	350	10	15	150
3.0	1200	1200	300	18	15	150
3.0	1200	1200	300	18	15	150
3.0	800	800	300	18	15	150
3.0	800	800	300	18	15	150
3.0	800	800	300	10	15	150
+ 1.0	+ 400	+ 400	+ 150	h	+ 5	+ 25
+ 1.0	+ 400	+ 400	+ 150	h	+ 10	+ 50

g The RDA for vitamin B12 in infants is based on average concentration of the vitamin in human milk. The allowances after weaning are based on energy intake (as recommended by the American Academy of Pediatrics) and consideration of other factors such as intestinal absorption.

h The increased requirement during pregnancy cannot be met by the iron content of habitual American diets nor by the existing iron stores of many women; therefore, the use of 30-60 mg of supplemental iron is recommended. Iron needs during lactation are not substantially different from those of non-pregnant women, but continued supplementation of the mother for 2-3 months after parturition is advisable in order to replenish stores depleted by pregnancy.

Table II
Recommended Dietary Allowances, Revised 1980

Estimated safe and adequate daily dietary intakes
of selected vitamins and minerals[a]

| | Vitamins | | | |
Age (years)	Vitamin K (μg)	Biotin (μg)	Pantothenic Acid (mg)	Copper (mg)
Infants				
0-0.5	12	35	2	0.5-0.7
0.5-1	10-20	50	3	0.7-1.0
Children and Adolescents				
1-3	15-30	65	3	1.0-1.5
4-6	20-40	85	3-4	1.5-2.0
7-10	30-60	120	4-5	2.0-2.5
11 +	50-100	100-200	4-7	2.0-3.0
Adults	70-140	100-200	4-7	2.0-3.0

[a] Because there is less information on which to base allowances, these figures are not given in the main table of the RDA and are provided here in the form of ranges of recommended intakes.

[b] Since the toxic levels for many trace elements may be only several times usual intakes, the upper levels for the trace elements given in this table should not be habitually exceeded.

Table II (continued)
Recommended Dietary Allowances, Revised 1980
Food and Nutrition Board, National Academy of
Sciences—National Research Council, Washington, D.C.

Trace Elements[b]				
Manganese (mg)	Fluoride (mg)	Chromium (mg)	Selenium (mg)	Molybdenum (mg)
0.5-0.7	0.1-0.5	0.01-0.04	0.01-0.04	0.03-0.06
0.7-1.0	0.2-1.0	0.02-0.06	0.02-0.06	0.04-0.08
1.0-1.5	0.5-1.5	0.02-0.08	0.02-0.08	0.05-0.1
1.5-2.0	1.0-2.5	0.03-0.12	0.03-0.12	0.06-0.15
2.0-3.0	1.5-2.5	0.05-0.2	0.05-0.2	0.1-0.3
2.5-5.0	1.5-2.5	0.05-0.2	0.05-0.2	0.15-0.5
2.5-5.0	1.5-4.0	0.05-0.2	0.05-0.2	0.15-0.5

	Electrolytes		
Age (years)	Sodium (mg)	Potassium (mg)	Chloride (mg)
Infants			
0-0.5	115-350	350-925	275-700
0.5-1	250-750	425-1275	400-1200
Children and Adolescents			
1-3	325-975	550-1650	500-1500
4-6	450-1350	775-2325	700-2100
7-10	600-1800	1000-3000	925-2775
11+	900-2700	1525-4575	1400-4200
Adults	1100-3300	1875-5625	1700-5100

Table III
Mean Heights and Weights and
Recommended Energy Intake[a]
Recommended Dietary Allowances, Revised 1980

Age (years)	Weight (kg)	(lbs)	Height (cm)	(in)	Energy Needs (with range) (kcal)	(MJ)
Infants						
0.0-0.5	6	13	60	24	kg × 115 (95-145)	kg × .48
0.5-1.0	9	20	71	28	kg × 105 (80-135)	kg × .44
Children						
1-3	13	29	90	35	1300 (900-1800)	5.5
4-6	20	44	112	44	1700 (1300-2300)	7.1
7-10	28	62	132	52	2400 (1650-3300)	10.1
Males						
11-14	45	99	157	62	2700 (2000-3700)	11.3
15-18	66	145	176	69	2800 (2100-3900)	11.8
19-22	70	154	178	70	2900 (2500-3300)	12.2
23-50	70	154	178	70	2700 (2300-3100)	11.3
51-75	70	154	178	70	2400 (2000-2800)	10.1
76+	70	154	178	70	2050 (1650-2450)	8.6
Females						
11-14	46	101	157	62	2200 (1500-3000)	9.2
15-18	55	120	163	64	2100 (1200-3000)	8.8
19-22	55	120	163	64	2100 (1700-2500)	8.8

Table III (continued)
Mean Heights and Weights and Recommended Energy Intake[a]
Recommended Dietary Allowances, Revised 1980

Age (years)	Weight (kg)	(lbs)	Height (cm)	(in)	Energy Needs (with range) (kcal)	(MJ)
Females						
23-50	55	120	163	64	2000 (1600-2400)	8.4
51-75	55	120	163	64	1800 (1400-2200)	7.6
76+	55	120	163	64	1600 (1200-2000)	6.7
Pregnancy					+300	
Lactation					+500	

[a] The data in this table have been assembled from the observed median heights and weights of children shown in Table I, together with desirable weights for adults given in Table II for the mean heights of men (70 inches) and women (64 inches) between the ages of 18 and 34 years as surveyed in the U.S. population (HEW/NCHS data).

The energy allowances for the young adults are for men and women doing light work. The allowances for the two older groups represent mean energy needs over these age spans, allowing for a 2% decrease in basal (resting) metabolic rate per decade and a reduction in activity of 200 kcal/day for men and women between 51 and 75 years, 500 kcal for men over 75 years and 400 kcal for women over 75. The customary range of daily energy output is shown for adults in parentheses, and is based on a variation in energy needs of ±400 kcal at any one age (Garrow, 1978), emphasizing the wide range of energy intakes appropriate for any group of people.

Energy allowances for children through age 18 are based on median energy intakes of children of these ages followed in longitudinal growth studies. The values in parentheses are 10th and 90th percentiles of energy intake, to indicate the range of energy consumption among children of these ages.

Eating Right Is Up to You

The "Basic Four" Food Group Plan
A Recommended Daily Guide

	Number of Servings	Portion Size
Meat– Protein Group	2	A serving = 2-3 oz cooked meat, fish, or chicken, ¼ cup tuna, 2 eggs, 4 tbsp peanut butter, 1 cup dry peas or beans (cooked), ½ cup nuts.
Milk–Dairy Group	2/adults 4/teenagers 3/children	Foods made from milk contribute part of the nutrients supplied by a serving of milk. A serving = 8 oz milk, 8 oz yogurt, 1½ cups cottage cheese, 2 cups ice cream, 1 cup milk pudding, 1-2 oz cheese.
Bread– Cereal/ Grain Group	4	A serving = 1 slice bread, ½ cup cooked cereal, 1 oz ready-to-eat cereal, ½ cup cooked rice, grits, macaroni, or spaghetti. Whole grain or enriched breads and cereals are recommended.

The "Basic Four" Food Group Plan
A Recommended Daily Guide

	Number of Servings	Portion Size
Fruits— Vegetables Group	4	A serving = ½ cup fruit, vegetable, or juice, 1 medium piece of fruit. Dark green, leafy, or orange vegetables and fruit are recommended three or four times weekly. Citrus fruit is recommended daily.
Others		Fats, oils, sweets, soft drinks, and alcohol contribute calories but do not replace foods from the "Basic Four" groups.

Sample of Nutrition Information Panel
The sample panel below was taken from a loaf of wheat bread.

Nutrition Information per serving
Serving size: 1 ounce (Approx. 1 slice)
Servings per pkg.: 16

	Per 1 oz. serving
Calories	70 grams
Protein	3 grams
Carbohydrates	13 grams
Fat	1
Cholesterol	Below 5 milligrams
Sodium	140 milligrams

Percentage of U.S. Recommended Daily Allowance (U.S. RDA)

	Per 1 oz. serving
Protein	4
Vitamin A	0
Vitamin C	0
Thiamin	8
Riboflavin	4
Niacin	6
Calcium	4
Iron	6

The U.S. RDA for Adults and Children Over Four

Nutrients that *must* be included in Nutrition Information panel:

Nutrient	U.S. RDA
Protein	65 g*
Vitamin C	60 mg
Vitamin A	5000 IU
Thiamine**	1.5 mg
Riboflavin	1.7 mg
Niacin	20 mg
Calcium	1 g
Iron	18 mg

Nutrients that *may* be included in Nutrition Information panel:

Nutrient	U.S. RDA
Vitamin D	400 IU
Vitamin E	30 IU
Vitamin B_6	2 mg
Folacin	0.4 mg
Vitamin B_{12}	6 μg
Biotin	0.3 mg
Pantothenic acid	10 mg
Phosphorus	1000 mg
Iodine	150 μg
Zinc	15 mg
Copper	2 mg
Magnesium	400 mg

* The value for protein may vary, depending upon the quality of protein in a specific food.

** The Food and Drug Administration uses the spelling "thiamine" rather than the more common spelling "thiamin."

Chapter 2

The Story of Vitamins

With all the talk about the importance of vitamins to good nutrition, it's time to ask "What *are* vitamins?" Vitamins are organic substances that are necessary in very small amounts to maintain normal metabolism in the body.

The word *vitamin* was coined as *vitamine* in 1912 by Dr. Casimir Funk, a Polish chemist working at the Lister Institute in London, and is derived from *vita*, meaning "life," and *amine*, referring to a class of nitrogen-containing organic compounds. At the time, Dr. Funk was investigating thiamin—vitamin B_1—which *really is* an amine. Later it was learned that not all of the vitamins were amines, so the final *e* in *vitamine* was dropped. The word, *vitamin*, however, still reflects the vital life-giving importance of these substances.

The words "in very small amounts" included in the definition of vitamins serve to distinguish them from the other classes of essential organic compounds. For example, proteins, fats, and carbohydrates are also organic substances, but we require them in considerably greater quantities. Vitamins are measured in milligrams (mg) and micrograms (µg), in contrast to proteins, fats, and carbohydrates, which are measured in grams (g). If you remember your mini-math lesson from the last chapter, 1 milligram = $\frac{1}{1,000}$ of a gram, 1 microgram = $\frac{1}{1,000,000}$ of a gram, and a gram is about the mass of a paper clip. If you think these extremely tiny amounts sound insignificant and that you can probably do all right without them, just remember the British sailors who developed scurvy on those long ocean voyages. Then you'll realize just how *absolutely vital* these minute quantities really are.

In the definition of vitamins, we also stated that they're *organic*. As such, they can be easily destroyed, oxidized, or changed in molecular form or shape. In our bodies, this quality is helpful since we may need to alter the form of a vitamin to make it more useful to us during certain body processes. In our foods, however, this same quality makes it possible for us to accidently reduce their vitamin content by improper handling, storing, or cooking.

We've only officially known about the presence of vitamins since Dr. Funk's research in 1912. Since that time, 13 vitamins have been identified. The last one to be isolated was vitamin B_{12} in the late 1940s.

As each vitamin was discovered, it was given a letter designation assigned in alphabetical order. It turned out, however, that some of the vitamins were actually composed of several substances. The compound called vitamin B, for example, was found to be a group of compounds, each of which is now given a numerical subscript in addition to the letter B. So we now have vitamin B_1, vitamin B_2, vitamin B_6, and so forth. Although vitamins' alphabetical designations are still in common use, they are also referred to by their chemical names.

You've probably heard the phrase *essential vitamins*. The term *essential* here means that these substances cannot be manufactured by the body and *must,* therefore, be supplied in our diet. As with any rule, there are always exceptions. The body *does* produce small amounts of riboflavin (vitamin B_1), biotin, and vitamin K, but in such negligible quantities that we still need additional quantities from the foods we eat.

The body is also capable of manufacturing certain other vitamins if it is supplied with the proper raw materials. For example, plant foods such as fruits and vegetables don't actually contain vitamin A, but instead have vitamin A activity. In other words, they contain substances which we can convert to vitamin A. Those substances are carotenes—the group of yellow-orange compounds which are present in and give the characteristic color to such vegetables and fruits as carrots, squash, and cantaloupes. For this reason, carotenes are known as precursors of vitamin A and are sometimes called provitamin A.

We have a provitamin D in our skin. The conversion to vitamin D takes place when the skin is exposed to sunlight—which explains why vitamin D is often called the sunshine vitamin. Generally, though, the amount produced in this way is too small to meet our bodies' needs, and a dietary source must still be supplied.

Because of the reliance on diet to fulfill our requirements of these vitamins, even vitamins A and D are classified as essential. The table on page 38 will help you identify the 13 essential vitamins and the chemical names by which they are known.

Vitamins are additionally classified by solubility. Those that dissolve in fat are classified as fat-soluble vitamins and they include vitamins A, D, E, and K. Those that dissolve in water are called water-soluble vitamins and they include biotin, folic acid, niacin, pantothenic acid, B_1, B_2, B_6, B_{12}, and vitamin C. Information about each of the 13 vitamins is provided in the vitamin sections of this book.

So Much From So Little

Many vitamins, especially those of the B-complex group, act as coenzymes—that is, small molecules that are attached to enzymes. An enzyme is an organic catalyst—a substance that regulates the speed of a chemical reaction without being used up or changed in that reaction. To our bodies, this means enzymes can be used over and over again to control specific reactions. Those vitamins that act as coenzymes can also be used by the body repeatedly. This fact helps to explain why only small amounts of these essential nutrients are needed. However, these vitamins are also water soluble and are, therefore, ex-

Continued on page 39

The Story of Vitamins

Vitamins and Their Chemical Names

Vitamin	Chemical Name
A	carotenoids; beta-carotene; retinol; vitamin A acetate; vitamin A palmitate
B_1	thiamin; thiamin hydrochloride; thiamin mononitrate
B_2	riboflavin; riboflavin-5'-phosphate; sodium riboflavin phosphate; disodium riboflavin phosphate
Niacin (B_3)	nicotinic acid; nicotinamide; niacinamide
B_6	pyridoxine hydrochloride
B_{12}	cobalamin; cyanocobalamin; cyanocobalamin concentrate
C	ascorbic acid; sodium ascorbate; erythorbic acid (isoascorbic acid)
D	cholecalciferol; calciferol; ergocalciferol
E	tocopherol; alpha tocopherol; alpha tocopheryl acetate; alpha tocopheryl acid succinate
K	naphthoquinone; menadione (K_3); phylloquinone (K_1, phytonadione) menaquinone (K_2)
Biotin	biotin
Folacin	folic acid; folate
Pantothenic acid	panthenol; calcium pantothenate

Continued from page 37
creted in the urine. Since they may be eliminated or otherwise broken down or changed by the body as necessary for certain metabolic processes, the body still needs a regular supply of these and the other essential vitamins to replace those lost or destroyed.

Vitamin Deficiency

When the amount of a nutrient in the diet or the total "body pool" of a nutrient is only marginally adequate, the condition is called a "subclinical deficiency." Biochemical and metabolic changes begin to take place, and an individual with this condition is considered to be at "risk" of a vitamin deficiency. Outward signs of a deficiency are not apparent, but symptoms can develop rapidly if the intake of this nutrient suddenly drops or if the person's nutrient requirement suddenly increases due to the impact of stress on the body's chemical makeup.

Identification of subclinical vitamin deficiency can be confirmed only by laboratory tests. Such tests include measurement of the amount of the vitamin in the blood and the amount of its breakdown products excreted in the urine. In some instances, metabolic derivatives of a vitamin are measured. In other cases, certain compounds tend to accumulate when the vitamin necessary for their further metabolism is in low supply. The amount of these compounds in the blood or urine is indicative of the vitamin status of the individual. It is also possible to measure the activity of certain enzymes which require vitamins as coenzymes. For example, the enzyme known as transketolase (present in red blood cells) has a below-normal degree of activity when the supply of the vitamin thiamin, its coenzyme, is limited. When such a lack is identified, dietary changes or even vitamin supplements may be necessary.

Fortunately, severe vitamin deficiencies are less widespread today than in earlier days, but they do exist, especially in areas of the world where malnutrition is prevalent.

Vitamin Toxicity

An overdose of a vitamin can be as serious as a deficiency. Large doses of vitamins have been shown to have harmful effects on the body. Fat-soluble vitamins, for example, are stored in body fat and used up as needed. The greater the intake, the greater the storage. The body, however, needs only tiny amounts of these vitamins to function properly. If too much is stored, serious consequences can result. Documented cases of toxicity, or excesses of vitamin A and D, have been reported. (For details, see the profiles devoted to these vitamins.)

Water-soluble vitamins are not stored in large amounts in the body. That's why we need a more constant supply of this group of vitamins. Normally, if too much is taken, the excess is excreted through the urine. Because of this, it was once believed that a person could not take in a dangerous amount of water-soluble vitamins. Yet, it has been shown that large quantities of vitamin C and some of the B vitamins have resulted in toxic effects.

High doses of vitamins can actually create vitamin imbalances. Large amounts of one vitamin can conceivably cause deficiencies of another. For example, animal studies have shown that high doses of vitamin E may adversely affect the status of vitamin K.

Hypervitaminosis is the clinical term for a vitamin overdose. It must be remembered that the danger of this condition exists whenever large doses—*megadoses*—of vitamins are consumed. For more information about this, refer to chapter 4 on megavitamin therapy.

Therapeutic Use and Vitamins as Drugs

There are many situations where vitamin intakes may need to be increased. For example, extra vitamins may be needed during periods of growth and development from infancy to the end of puberty. Since they're eating for two (or more), most pregnant women need extra nutrients. Vitamin supplementation may also be required when a person cannot consume a regular diet because of severe illness, surgery, or allergies. Vitamin requirements also increase for those taking birth control pills, those who are on very restrictive diets, and those who are taking drugs that may interfere with vitamin function or absorption. In rare instances, a person may be born with an inherited disorder requiring vitamin intakes that are quite different from those of a healthy individual. All of these situations need to be carefully evaluated and treated by a qualified physician.

Currently there is widespread promotion of "megavitamin therapy" or "orthomolecular therapy." Promotion is based on the premise that large doses of vitamins are useful for the prevention, treatment, or cure of many diseases. Although large doses of certain vitamins have been shown to be medically useful (as, for example, nicotinic acid—a form of niacin—in the reduction of blood-cholesterol levels), many other claims have been unsubstantiated by carefully controlled experimental studies.

Any possible drug-like action of a vitamin is unrelated to its nutritional function. A vitamin is not acting as a nutrient when taken in megadoses because the amount far exceeds that necessary to meet the body's nutritional requirements. Rather, as a megadose, the vitamin is being used as a drug. *Self-treatment of real or suspected diseases with massive doses of vitamins is potentially hazardous*. Not only does the danger of overdose exist, but self-diagnosis and self-treatment can only delay appropriate medical attention.

In addition, there is no nutritionally sound basis for using megadoses of vitamins as "insurance" against possible dietary shortages. There is no substitute for a proper diet. Supplements with vitamins in amounts much greater than those recommended by the RDA should not be used without proper medical supervision.

Vitaminlike Substances

Certain substances, although not considered true vitamins, closely resemble vitamins in their activity. They are commonly called vitaminlike substances. When listed in vitamin preparations, these substances are usually footnoted with a phrase similar to this one: "Need in human nutrition has not been established."

The nutritional status and biological role of vitaminlike substances requires further research. At one time choline, inositol and para-aminobenzoic acid (PABA) were thought to be vitamins. It was later discovered that each of these could be synthesized in the body, and a lack of them did not cause deficiency symptoms. Therefore, they do not meet the requirements of an essential vitamin.

Claims have been made that PABA will protect against sunburn. PABA *is* used as an ingredient in some sunscreens applied to the skin, but taking PABA internally will not prevent sunburn. It's also been suggested that PABA will prevent gray hair. When some animals are deprived of PABA, their dark fur loses its pigment. However, PABA cannot reverse or prevent graying in humans. Once a person's hair has turned gray, nothing short of a bottle of dye will restore his or her natural color.

Other vitaminlike substances include: bioflavonoids (often sold in combination with vitamin C); carnitine (sometimes called vitamin B-T); coenzyme Q; and lipoic acid.

The Story of Vitamins

Current widespread promotion of vitaminlike supplements for the treatment or cure of serious diseases is not supported by scientific evidence. Vitaminlike substances are not essential for good health. Only the 13 vitamins discussed in the following chapters are considered essential in the human diet.

Well, we've come to the end of our general vitamin story. Following a chapter on vitamin supplements, and another on megavitamin therapy, you'll be ready to dive right into the individual vitamin profiles to discover the reasons why these nutrients really are so vital to life.

Chapter 3

Vitamin Supplements

Vitamin supplements are available in many varieties—as liquids, tablets, or time-release capsules. Different forms may be natural or synthetic, chewable or nonchewable, regular or fruit-flavored. They may contain only one vitamin or multiple vitamins and even nonvitamin substances. Dosages may vary widely from one supplement to another, from relatively low to extremely high quantities.

Confusion and misinformation surrounds the use of supplements. People hear stories that our food supply is being robbed of its nutritional value, and that it's difficult to get the required vitamins through our daily diets alone. Promoters of vitamin supplements encourage these stories with such expressions as *"just to be sure* you get all the vitamins you need." In addition, supplements—especially in massive doses —are being promoted for the prevention and cure of diseases totally unrelated to known deficiencies.

Even with all our knowledge of vitamins, the notion that vitamins are endowed with miraculous powers still persists. This idea, combined with a misunderstanding about how vitamins work, leads many to believe that daily vitamin supplements are essential for good health.

Making sense out of all this may seem like an impossible task. Not so, however. Read on. You'll be surprised to find yourself cutting through the tangled web that has woven its way around the topic of vitamin supplementation.

Vitamin Status—USA

Full-blown vitamin deficiency diseases are seldom seen in the United States today. Most practicing doctors have never seen a case of scurvy, beriberi, pellagra, or rickets. Those deficiencies that do occur can be traced to poverty, child abuse or neglect, ignorance or indifference about food selection, or adoption of bizarre eating habits. Although vitamin deficiencies are rarely seen, this doesn't necessarily mean, however, that the nutrition and vitamin status of the population is completely satisfactory.

A dietary lack of a vitamin produces a continuum of effects. As body tissues lose their vitamin reserves, metabolic reactions that require the vitamin are adversely affected, and symptoms begin to appear. As we said earlier, the stages prior to development of readily apparent symptoms have been characterized as "subclinical deficiency." This condition may or may not impair overall health, but it definitely represents a state of nutritional risk.

Vitamin Supplements

The vitamin status of more than 60,000 Americans of all ages was evaluated during the Ten-State Nutrition Survey (TSNS) between the years 1968 and 1970 and conducted by the Nutrition Program of the United States Public Health Service. Most of the participants in the survey were from low-income populations.

The original plan for the survey did not include evaluation of status for all of the essential vitamins, and physical examinations did not reveal obvious symptoms of vitamin deficiency. Yet, blood and urine analysis showed that many of those included in the survey population were at risk levels. That is, they were in danger of developing vitamin deficiency. Among those surveyed, Mexican-Americans in Texas had a major problem with respect to vitamin A. Young people in general had unsatisfactorily low blood plasma vitamin A values. Riboflavin status was poor among blacks and among young people of all ethnic groups. (Vitamins now known to be important, like vitamin B_6 and folacin, were not studied and neither were many important minerals.) The major nutrition problem, however, was that of iron intake and associated iron deficiency anemia.

The dietary studies tended to correlate with the findings of clinical and biochemical examinations for the study population. For example, individuals with low blood plasma vitamin A concentrations also consumed relatively low amounts of the vitamin. Analysis of food intake records indicated that unsatisfactory nutritional status was more a function of the quantity of food available than of the quality of the diets. In other words, many people simply did not have enough to eat. This related to family income—the lower the income, the poorer the nutritional status.

In 1971–74, the National Center for Health Statistics conducted its first Health and Nutrition Examination Survey (HANES) with objectives and procedures similar to those of the TSNS. In the HANES study, however, the more than 20,000 people who were surveyed represented a broader cross-section of the American population. Participants were not concentrated in the low-income group. Again, nutrient deficiencies were found for vitamin A and iron, in addition to protein and calcium.

In 1977, HANES II was conducted as a follow-up to the first study. It attempted to determine if the low nutrient intakes found in HANES I would be reflected in the physical condition and laboratory test results of the subjects. Low lab values were found in some of the participants for such nutrients as protein, vitamin A, thiamin, riboflavin, and iron. Yet, not everyone with a low intake of a nutrient had low values. Investigators felt that some of those with low intakes were probably at the very beginning stages of deficiency.

In 1977–78, the United States Department of Agriculture conducted the Nationwide Food Consumption Survey. Like earlier surveys, it was found that dietary adequacy was related to income. A surprise finding was that although Americans were becoming more obese (probably as a result of inactivity), they were not consuming large amounts of calories. This means, for example, that an average woman who stayed within the calorie allowance needed to maintain her weight would not be getting the recommended amounts of many nutrients. The survey also indicated that for vitamins A, C, and B_6, and the minerals calcium, iron, and magnesium, about ⅓ of the participants were getting only 70 percent or less of the RDA. Another finding of this survey was that most Americans were eating similar amounts and kinds of foods—high in fat, sugar, and cholesterol. This drew a great deal of attention to the need for nutrition education for all.

Unfortunately, findings from nutrition surveys are used in misleading ways to promote the sale of vitamin supplements. Advertisements for vitamins often include statements like "Surveys show that a large number of people in our country don't get all the vitamins they need." The implication is that these people need vitamin supplements. Statements of this sort are made with no qualification or reference to the factors responsible for the low vitamin intakes.

It should be remembered that most of the country's nutrition problems could be corrected by increasing food supplies to those in need, or by improving food selections or eating habits.

Who Needs Vitamin Supplements?

"Do I need vitamin supplements?" you may ask. No firm answer is possible without a thorough investiga-

Vitamin Supplements

tion of your individual eating habits, lifestyle, and all the other factors that affect the intake and use of the nutrients in your daily diet.

Actual vitamin deficiencies due to a faulty diet or appearing as the result of some disease condition should be treated with appropriate vitamin supplements. In either case, diagnosis of a deficiency should be made by a qualified physician. If precipitated by disease, the disease must be treated. Treatment is conducted on an individual basis with knowledge of the disease and its effect on vitamin status.

Vitamin supplement therapy for treatment of diseases unrelated to vitamin deficiency is effective in a mere few instances. Unfortunately, the consumer is constantly exposed to the promotion of vitamins as wonder drugs. Such promotion is often motivated more by money than by health concerns, and unfettered by constraints imposed by medicine, science, or ethics.

Prevention of diseases other than deficiency diseases through the use of vitamin supplements is extremely difficult to prove or disprove. A person who takes vitamins and does not develop a certain disease often attributes his or her good fortune to the supplement. But, without a direct connection between the supplement and a particular disease, the mere fact that a person doesn't get the disease is not sufficient evidence to warrant the use of a supplement for the purpose of prevention. Many people end up taking vitamin supplements as a type of "nutrition insurance." They don't know what their vitamin status is, and they don't know the amount of vitamins present in the foods they eat, so they use vitamin supplements "just to be sure."

Nutritionists generally agree that people can get all the vitamins they need from foods, if the right ones are eaten. However, they may not argue with the use of supplements for extra "insurance" as long as they're taken in amounts not exceeding the RDAs. Nutrition experts, such as those of the American Dietetic Association, do not support the use of supplements containing megadoses of vitamins.

If you want to know if you really *need* to take vitamin supplements, CONSUMER GUIDE® recommends that you consult your doctor. Together, the two of you can can determine your nutritional needs based on your present state of health and any other pertinent circumstances.

Supplements Are Not Substitutes for the Real Thing

Some people think that as long as they take vitamin supplements they don't need to worry about how or what they eat. Not so. *To ensure good nutrition and good health, all essential nutrients, not just vitamins, must be supplied in adequate amounts.* Nutrients are all part of a team, and vitamins are just one of the players. *Vitamin supplements are not substitutes for good food.* They should not be used as an excuse for making poor food choices or having bad eating habits.

Vitamin Supplements

Vitamins and Dieters

Diets that include a variety of foods from the Basic Four Food Groups will usually supply an adequate amount of vitamins. In attempting to lose weight, however, many people are following weight-reduction diets that do not include or give proper emphasis to the Basic Four. (If you need a quick review of the Basic Four, see chapter 1, titled "Eating Right Is Up to You.") Even without restricting the types of foods you eat, if you cut down on calories, you automatically take in less food. Consequently, there is concern that vitamin intakes may be less than desirable among calorie-conscious people. In this situation, vitamin supplements *may* provide a bit of insurance against possible deficiency. However, your general state of health should be evaluated by your doctor before you begin a weight-reduction diet, any exercise program that may accompany the diet plan, and any vitamin supplementation. Medical supervision during this time can prove to be a wise investment.

Vitamins and the Elderly

There is growing concern among nutrition experts that the vitamin status of elderly people may be threatened by inadequate or inappropriate diets. Both the Ten-State Nutrition Survey (TSNS) and the Health and Nutrition Examination Survey (HANES) suggest that many older people are eating diets containing less than ⅔ of the RDAs for many vitamins and minerals.

Vitamin Supplements

In an ongoing study of over 700 senior citizens in the Boston area, researchers are finding that the diets of these older Americans are providing less than 2/3 of the recommended dietary allowances for such nutrients as vitamins B_6, B_{12}, and D, folic acid, zinc, calcium, and magnesium. Why are their diets providing less than adequate amounts of these and other important nutrients?

Many elderly people do not eat well because of economic problems, loneliness, physical handicaps, and/or reduced mobility. Many also cut down on the amounts of food eaten to avoid becoming overweight. However, by cutting down on calories, for whatever reason, nutrient intakes are decreased, and deficiencies can occur.

For the elderly, daily multivitamin/mineral supplements that supply 100 percent of the RDAs may be indicated. A doctor's supervision in both the choice and dosage of these supplements is necessary to ensure proper use. But, it should be noted that use of supplements can never substitute for foods. Supplements lack carbohydrates, fats, proteins, and many other important nutrients. Therefore, every attempt should be made by older persons to eat a balanced diet whether supplements are taken or not.

Vitamins for Pregnant Women, Infants, and Children

Vitamin supplements are almost routinely prescribed for pregnant women, since pregnancy increases the need for vitamins. The use of supplements provides a certain degree of assurance that vitamin requirements will be met.

An infant fed breast milk may not get enough vitamin D. On the other hand, an infant fed evaporated milk formulas will get only small amounts of vitamin C. Consequently, pediatricians frequently prescribe supplements containing vitamins D and C for babies. Usually in liquid form, the supplement, which generally contains vitamin A as well, can be added to formulas, soft foods, or squirted directly into the mouth. As with any vitamin supplement, it should be used only according to directions.

Chewable vitamin supplements are popular for young children. They're available in a variety of flavors, sizes and shapes—animals, flowers, and popular cartoon characters—to interest the child into taking them. However, this very appeal, their candy-like appearance and taste, has caused concern about possible overuse. Even though they're sold with child-proof bottle caps, there have been many reports of poisoning from the consumption of large numbers of chewable children's vitamins. *These, as well as any other vitamin-mineral supplements or drugs, must be kept out of the reach of children.*

A child, like an adult, can ordinarily acquire all the vitamins he or she needs from food. Nutritionists emphasize the importance of introducing a child to the Basic Four Food Groups as well as to good eating habits in early stages of development. Though doctors may recommend the use of supplements during a child's formative years, supplements *should not be used as an excuse for allowing a child to develop bad eating habits.*

Synthetic Versus Natural

If you're going to use supplements, here's something to think about. Vitamins that are present in foods are considered to be natural. Those that are created in a laboratory are referred to as synthetic. Both are sold in supplement form.

Synthetic vitamins are copies of the original natural vitamin that was isolated from food. They're readily available, usually cheaper in price than natural vitamin supplements, and their potency can be controlled.

Vitamins used to enrich or fortify foods and those present in most supplements are synthetic—products of the laboratory rather than nature. Vitamin C was the first vitamin synthesized in 1933.

What you need to remember as a consumer is that a vitamin is a vitamin regardless of its source. A vitamin made by a plant is essentially identical to one made by a drug company. So far as we know, our bodies cannot tell the difference.

Checking the Label

The following sample labels illustrate the kind of information that you'll probably find on vitamin sup-

Vitamin Supplements

plement containers. The front panel shows the brand name of the product (manufacturer's name will appear here or elsewhere on the label), the kind of supplement, and the number of tablets or capsules in the container. Types of supplements include single nutrients, multivitamins, and multivitamin/multiminerals. They're available in a variety of potencies from therapeutic doses which contain amounts many times greater than the U.S. RDA, to doses which supply only U.S. RDA levels or less.

The label also gives directions for use (e.g. "One tablet daily"). The vitamins and/or minerals in the supplement are listed next as "Percent of the U.S. RDA for Adults and Children Four or More Years of Age." Supplements prepared for infants and children under age four, or for pregnant or lactating (nursing) women, list the percent of the U.S. RDA for these specific groups. We recommend that you select a preparation that provides vitamins in amounts approximating 100 percent of the U.S. RDAs and avoid those with amounts in excess of the U.S. RDAs. To be sure of your choice, check with your doctor. A supplement like the one illustrated would be a good choice.

All but one of the vitamins in our sample are provided in amounts equal to 100 percent of the U.S. RDA. For vitamin E, only 50 percent of the U.S. RDA is furnished. That's because the U.S. RDAs were derived from the 1968 revision of the Food and Nutrition Board's Recommended Daily Dietary Allowances when the adult RDA for vitamin E was 30 IU.

Continued on page 58

Sample Portions of a Vitamin Supplement Label

Front Panel

VITA-SURE*
MULTIVITAMIN SUPPLEMENT

For adults and children
4 or more years of age

100 tablets

Wishing-You-Well Vitamin Company*

Contents Panel

Directions: Take one tablet daily. Each tablet contains:

Vitamin	Quantity	Percent of U.S. RDA
Vitamin A	5,000 IU	100
Vitamin E	15 IU	50
Vitamin C	60 mg	100
Folic Acid	0.4 mg	100
Thiamin	1.5 mg	100
Riboflavin	1.7 mg	100
Niacin	20 mg	100
Vitamin B_6	2 mg	100
Vitamin B_{12}	6 µg	100
Vitamin D	400 IU	100
Pantothenic Acid	10 mg	100

Expiration date—July 1991

*These names are used for purpose of illustration only. They are not meant to represent an actual product or company.

Vitamin Supplements

Continued from page 56

The amounts of the nutrients are usually given in milligrams (mg), micrograms (μg) and international units (IU). Recall that a milligram is $1/1,000$ of a gram, while a microgram is $1/1,000$ of a milligram or $1/1,000,000$ of a gram, and there are 28 grams in an ounce. The term *international unit* refers to the amount of the vitamin that will cure deficiency symptoms in a laboratory animal. This term is no longer used on the RDA tables but is still used on labels.

The contents panel also includes: *names* of the vitamins and/or minerals included in the supplement; *ingredients as the source or form of each vitamin and/or mineral* (listed in descending order by weight); *the chemical name* of each nutrient (A table of the various chemical names used for vitamins can be found on page 38.); *ingredients used to form the tablet or capsule* (For example, corn starch may be used as a filler, binder, or disintegrating agent, propyl paraben used as a coating, and vanillin as a flavoring agent.); a *warning* (e.g. "Keep out of the reach of children."); an *expiration date*, which is the date when the supplement should no longer be used (Taking a vitamin past this date is not dangerous, but its potency may be reduced. However, if there's any change in color, taste, smell, or appearance, you should discard the supplement. Minerals, on the other hand, are very stable and can be used for an indefinite period.); and *storage instructions*. Vitamins should be stored in their original container, in a cool, dry place. The kitchen and bathroom are not the best places, as the heat and humidity hasten deterioration.

Continued on page 60

Sample Portions of a Vitamin Supplement Label

Front Panel

MOTHER NATURE'S TABLE† VITAMINS AND
MINERALS from NATURAL SOURCES plus
Additional Natural Ingredients
100 tablets
Be-Well Vitamin Company†

Contents Panel

Directions: Take six tablets daily. Each six (6) tablets contain:

Vitamin	Quantity	Percent of U.S. RDA*
Vitamin A (fish liver oil)	10,000 IU	200
Vitamin D (fish liver oil)	400 IU	100
Vitamin E	100 IU	333
Vitamin C (natural vitamin C and rose hips)	300 mg	500
Folic Acid	200 μg	50
Vitamin B_1 (yeast concentrate)	10 mg	666
Vitamin B_6 (yeast concentrate)	10 mg	588
Niacin (yeast concentrate)	10 mg	50
Vitamin B_6	1 mg	50
Vitamin B_{12} activity (cobalamin concentrate)	25 μg	417
Biotin	0.15 mg	50
Pantothenic Acid	5 mg	50
Choline (yeast concentrate)	24 mg	**

*U.S. Recommended Daily Allowance (U.S. RDA) for adults and children four or more years of age.

**No U.S. RDA has been established for this nutrient.

†These names are used for purpose of illustration only. They are not meant to represent an actual product or company.

Vitamin Supplements

Continued from page 58
The front panel and contents panel on page 59 is a sample label from a "natural" supplement. The front panel shows that it's a vitamin/mineral supplement from natural sources. The label might also say, "Made with food vitamins and food minerals." The term "natural" might also mean the vitamins and minerals are in a natural base with no artificial additives. In this case, the vitamins may be synthetic, but the other ingredients come from natural sources.

The amounts of the vitamins and minerals are given for comparison with the label shown previously. The actual label for such a natural supplement would also include a list of ingredients or "other compounds" in the formulation (such as the vitaminlike substance PABA).

Some of the natural sources for the vitamins are shown as fish liver oil, yeast concentrate, and rose hips. The vitamins represent 50 to 666 percent of the U.S. RDAs. Choline is included in the list, although it is not recognized as an essential vitamin, and no U.S. RDA has been established for it. Calcium and phosphorus, the two minerals included in this product, came from tricalcium phosphate, a substance which is a natural constituent of plants and animals. Calcium and phosphorus are provided in only 4 and 7 percent of the U.S. RDA. If the tablets contained larger amounts of these minerals, they might be too large to swallow.

A variety of sources such as yeast, dried liver, fish liver oils, wheat germ oil, and bone marrow are used

to prepare natural supplements. It would be techni-
cally difficult to make a supplement with exactly 100
percent of the U.S. RDA from only natural sources
for all of the vitamins and minerals. And the safety
of such a product might be questionable. In the sample shown, many of the vitamins are provided at
levels that far exceed the U.S. RDAs, and that can
be dangerous. (See the individual vitamin profiles for
specific information.)

There is no evidence to prove that natural vitamins
are in any way superior to synthetic vitamins. In
addition, natural vitamins usually cost more (for
example, one brand of an all-natural vitamin costs
more than $1 a day when taken in the amount
suggested on the label). The label may suggest that
you're getting some important "extras." These "extras," however, are not dietary essentials. And, the
higher amounts of vitamins provided have no known
nutritional value and might actually be harmful.

How to Buy Vitamin Supplements

The cost of supplements varies widely from brand
to brand, from one retailer to another, and with the
number of daily doses per container. The quality varies,
too. This is especially true when vitamins come from
a local supplier, do not cross state lines, and are not
covered by Interstate Commerce regulations.

The cost of a supplement usually increases as the
numbers of doses in the package increase. The daily

Continued on page 63

Composition of Selected Natural Vitamin Supplements
Percent of U.S. RDA in amount recommended for daily use

	Mega Food	Nutri-Time	Natural Nutrivits	Sun Chlorella*
Vitamin A	300	500	200	35
Vitamin D	150	250	100	
Thiamin (B_1)	1,000	1,200	333	4
Riboflavin (B_2)	882	1,056	588	8
Vitamin B_6	750	625	300	2
Vitamin B_{12}	500	300	400	**
Vitamin C	833	500	250	**
Vitamin E	500	100	50	**
Vitamin K	**			
Niacin	450	300	100	4
Pantothenic Acid	600	300	50	**
Folic Acid	100	100		
Biotin	100	20		2
Inositol		***		
Choline		**	***	
Rutin			***	
Para-aminobenzoic Acid		***		
Bioflavonoids			***	
Calcium	25	75	13	6
Chromium	**			
Copper	30	50		**
Iodine	100	100	30	10
Magnesium	25	7.5		2
Manganese	**			

Composition of Selected Natural Vitamin Supplements (continued)
Percent of U.S. RDA in amount recommended for daily use

	Mega Food	Nutri-Time	Natural Nutrivits	Sun Chlorella*
Molybdenum	**			
Selenium	**			
Potassium	**			
Vanadium	**			
Zinc	100	100		15
Phosphorus		36	25	4
Iron		330		5
Cost per day	$.93– 1.35	$.12– .36	$.05	$1.00

Blank spaces indicate no information about that nutrient is provided.

*Sun Chlorella also contains 19 amino acids in varying amounts.

**Contains less than 2 percent of U.S. RDA.

***Indicates product contains substance, but that U.S. RDA and/or need in human nutrition has not been established: no nutritional claims made for it.

The costs per day of vitamin supplements listed in this table were based on East Coast prices in March 1988 and do not reflect a national average.

Continued from page 61
cost of a vitamin supplement will be less when a package of 250 tablets is purchased, in contrast to the daily cost of a supplement with only 60 tablets. The average cost per day of a multivitamin supplement providing 100 percent of the U.S. RDAs ranges from about three cents to slightly more than six cents, depending upon the brand and the retail outlet. If you decide to use a vitamin supplement, check labels to identify those with only 100 percent of the U.S.

Vitamin Supplements

RDAs, then make a cost comparison. Divide the cost per container by the number of daily doses (tablets, capsules, or liquid measure) to find the cost per day.

There are a number of supplements that, in addition to supplying vitamins at 100 percent of the U.S. RDAs, also include iron at 100 percent. These may cost slightly more per day than those containing only vitamins. The addition of other minerals or use of high potency doses also raises the price—in fact, may even double the cost of a single dose. Natural supplements, which usually contain both vitamins and minerals, may cost over $1 per day. (See the table on pages 62-63 for comparative contents and costs of several natural vitamin supplements.)

After this lengthy discussion on supplements, we hope that at least one important fact stays with you: It's all right to take supplements when they're called for, but *there's no real substitute for a well-balanced diet.*

Chapter 4

Megavitamin Therapy

We've all heard claims for megavitamin therapy. "You should take extra B vitamins when your body is under stress," they'll say, or "Schizophrenia can be controlled with large amounts of niacin" or even "You can eliminate the symptoms of menopause by taking lots of vitamin E."

Today, people are bombarded with claims for miracle cures by "megavitamin" therapy promoters who say that vitamin supplements (sometimes containing as much as several thousand percent of the U.S. RDA) are effective in treating many physical and mental disorders. Unfortunately, these claims have not been supported by controlled clinical studies.

Just *what is* megavitamin therapy? Megavitamin therapy is defined as the use of a vitamin in doses that are *ten or more times its recommended dietary allowance.* For example, the RDA for adult intake of vitamin C is 60 mg, so 600 mg or more of vitamin C would be considered a megavitamin dose.

Megavitamin Therapy

The idea that "if a little is good, a lot must be better" does not apply to vitamins. As we've discussed earlier, when you take in more of a vitamin than you need, the excess acts like a drug in the body, not like a vitamin. For this reason, you run the risk of experiencing harmful side effects just as you would by overdosing on a particular drug.

Whether vitamin/mineral supplements should be considered as drugs or as food supplements complicates the issue of their regulation. The Center for Food Safety and Applied Nutrition of the Food and Drug Administration (FDA) has the authority to limit the potency or composition of only those vitamin/mineral supplements considered to be food supplements for use in children and pregnant or nursing women. The FDA has authority only over the folic acid composition of food supplements to be used by other members of the population. All other vitamins found in food supplements are not regulated. Other divisions of the FDA have control over the vitamin/mineral supplements that are considered to be drugs, such as prenatal vitamins. The Federal Trade Commission and the FDA jointly control advertising of vitamin/mineral supplements. However, neither agency has effective supplement regulations. This means that supplement advertising is only minimally controlled. Development of needed regulations has been hampered by the lack of standard definitions necessary to categorize the supplements as either food or drugs.

Some people may be able to take megadoses of some vitamins without serious side effects. But, evidence of potential hazards associated with the intake of large doses of vitamins continues to grow. You will see references to this in the individual vitamin profiles.

When promoters of megavitamin therapy raise false hopes, they are little better than hawkers at a frontier medicine show. The book "Life Extension" by Durk Pearson and Sandy Shaw suggests that heart disease and cancer can be prevented or significantly delayed by taking megadoses of approximately 25 nutrient supplements daily. Jack Z. Yetiv, MD., Ph.D., in his book "Popular Nutritional Practices: A Scientific Appraisal," evaluates the Pearson-Shaw book and finds it to be " . . . extremely inaccurate; some of the recommendations in the book are potentially life-threatening." The references given in the Pearson-Shaw book *do not support the claims* that have been made, and at times even contradict them. This book is typical of the many books promoting megavitamin therapy. They tempt the public with false claims and false hopes, while in reality offering little more than unproven, often expensive regimens that may harm the user.

Those who believe in megavitamin therapy may develop serious guilt feelings when they think they might have protected a loved one from serious disease—had they "only known" sooner. The late nutrition author Adelle Davis made the unsupported claim that crib deaths could be prevented by breast-feeding and taking vitamin E. For a family who has lost a child to this untimely killer, statements like this can only add to what is already profound grief.

Megavitamin Therapy

The use of unsubstantiated megavitamin therapies to self-treat a disease may endanger a person's life if necessary medical treatment is delayed. *Large amounts of vitamins are not cure-alls*. As we've said before, again and again, large amounts can be very dangerous. Anything that is consumed can be poisonous if enough is taken. Vitamins are no different.

While vitamin supplements can cure a deficiency of a particular vitamin or vitamins, excess amounts of vitamins can interfere with medications or other vitamins, disrupt body functions, and can be toxic to the body.

So, what is a simple rule of thumb to remember about the use of vitamins? *DON'T OVERDOSE*.

Now, it's time to examine the individual vitamins one by one.

Chapter 5

Vitamin Profiles
Vitamin A:
Retinol

As far as vitamin A is concerned, the eyes have it. The essential nutrient known as vitamin A, or retinol, plays a vital role in vision. You'll learn about this and other important functions of vitamin A later in this chapter.

History

As indicated by its position at the head of the "vitamin alphabet," vitamin A was the first to be "found." It was discovered in the early 1900s after researchers recognized that a certain substance in animal fats and fish oils was necessary for the growth of young animals. Because it was found in animal fats, the substance was originally called *fat-soluble A*. Its name was soon changed to *vitamin A*.

Vitamin A includes several compounds that have similar biological activity. These compounds are retinol and the carotenes. Retinol is vitamin A as we know it—the natural form of the vitamin that's found in foods of animal origin. Carotenes are provitamins,

Vitamin A: Retinol

substances the body can use to manufacture a vitamin. They occur in foods of plant origin.

Function of Vitamin A

The most clearly defined role of vitamin A is the part it plays in vision, especially the ability to see in the dark. Metabolites of the vitamin combine with certain proteins to make visual pigments that help the eye adjust from bright to dim light. Vitamin A is used up in this process. If it's not replaced, night blindness results. In addition, the health of the eye itself depends on vitamin A. When there's a deficiency, the transparent coating of the eye (called the cornea) and the "whites" of the eye (called the conjunctiva) become dry. This condition is called *xerophthalmia*. If it continues unchecked, irreversible damage and blindness may follow. Vitamin A deficiency is a major cause of blindness in many parts of the world.

Vitamin A is also needed for normal growth and reproduction. Development of bones and teeth require a supply of this vitamin. Animal studies show that vitamin A is essential to normal sperm formation and to the maintenance of a healthy fetus.

Another important role of the vitamin involves the maintenance of healthy skin on all body surfaces inside and out, including the mucus membranes that line the gastrointestinal and respiratory tracts. In this way, vitamin A helps the body resist infection. Vitamin A may also be involved in the synthesis of steroid hormones.

Sources of Vitamin A

Vitamin A is found in foods of both plant and animal origin. Retinol, also called "preformed vitamin A," is the form present in animals. Carotenes, found in plants, are provitamins that can be converted to vitamin A in the body.

Liver is the single best food source of vitamin A. However, many experts recommend that liver should not be eaten more than once or twice a month because of the toxic substances it contains. (The toxins result from exposure of the animal to environmental pollutants. The longer the animal is alive, the greater the exposure. This means that the liver of a calf should contain less toxins and therefore, may be a healthier choice than the liver of a full-grown cow.) Egg yolk, cheese, whole milk, butter, fortified skim milk, and margarine are good sources. Red palm oil, used in cooking in many tropical countries, and fish liver oils, used as supplements, are rich in vitamin A. One tablespoon of cod liver oil contains 12,000 IU, more than twice the daily recommended intake for adults.

Orange and yellow fruits and vegetables have high vitamin A values because of the carotenes they contain. Generally, the darker the vegetable, the more carotene present. Carrots, for example, are especially good sources of carotene, and so they have high vitamin A value. Green, leafy vegetables like spinach also contain a lot of carotene, but the orange-yellow pigment is masked by the green pigment they pos-

Continued on page 75

Vitamin A: Retinol

Sources of Vitamin A

Food	Quantity	Percent of U.S. RDA
Beef liver, fried	2 ounces	605.60
Dandelion greens, raw	1 cup	504.00
Dandelion greens, cooked	1 cup	421.20
Sweet potatoes, canned	1 cup	340.00
Apricot halves; dried, uncooked	1 cup	327.00
Pumpkin, canned	1 cup	291.80
Spinach, cooked	1 cup	291.60
Spinach; canned, drained	1 cup	288.00
Sweet potatoes, boiled (peeled after boiling)	1 medium	232.20
Sweet potatoes, candied	1 potato	220.60
Collards, cooked	1 cup	205.20
Red hot peppers, dried (without seeds)	1 tablespoon	195.00
Cress; garden, raw	3 ½ ounces	186.00
Peas and carrots, frozen (boiled, drained)	3 ½ ounces	186.00
Kale; boiled, drained	1 cup	180.40
Sweet potatoes, baked (peeled after baking)	1 medium	178.20
Winter squash, baked (mashed)	1 cup	172.20
Apricots; dried, cooked, unsweetened (fruit and liquid)	1 cup	171.00
Turnip greens, cooked	1 cup	165.40
Kale, cooked (leaves and stems)	1 cup	162.80

Sources of Vitamin A (continued)

Food	Quantity	Percent of U.S. RDA
Mustard greens, cooked	1 cup	162.40
Beet greens; cooked, drained (leaves and stems)	1 cup	148.00
Cantaloupe	½ medium	130.80
Peaches; dried, uncooked	1 cup	124.80
Carrot, raw	1 whole	110.00
Cabbage; spoon or bok choy, cooked	1 cup	105.40
Apricots, canned in heavy syrup	1 cup	90.20
Broccoli, cooked, drained	1 medium stalk	90.00
Butter	½ cup	75.00
Margarine	½ cup	75.00
Peach halves; dried, cooked, unsweetened (fruit and liquid)	1 cup	65.80
Papayas, raw	1 cup (½-inch cubes)	63.80
Sweet potato pie	1 sector	62.40
Chicken pot pie, baked	1 pie (pre-bake weight, 8 ounces)	60.40
Plums, canned with syrup	1 cup	59.40
Vegetarian soups; canned, condensed (with equal amount water)	1 cup	58.80
Apricots, raw	3 apricots	57.80

Continued on next page

Vitamin A: Retinol

Sources of Vitamin A (continued)

Food	Quantity	Percent of U.S. RDA
Vegetable beef soup; canned, condensed (with equal amount water)	1 cup	54.00
Watermelon, raw	1 wedge (4 by 8 inches)	50.20
Minestrone soup; canned, condensed (with equal amount water)	1 cup	47.00
Beef and vegetable stew	1 cup	46.20
Tomatoes, canned (solids and liquid)	1 cup	43.40
Tomato juice, canned	1 cup	38.80
Sour cream	1 cup	38.60
Lettuce, cos or romaine	3½ ounces	38.00
Endive, curly (including escarole)	2 ounces	37.40
Beef pot pie, baked	1 pie (pre-bake weight, 8 ounces)	37.20
Prunes; dried, medium, cooked, unsweetened	1 cup	37.20
Crab, steamed	3 ounces	36.90
Palm oil	1 tablespoon	36.62
Swordfish, broiled with butter or margarine	3 ounces	35.00
Lake whitefish; stuffed, baked	3 ounces	34.00
Tomato-vegetable soup with noodles, dehydrated	1 package (2½ ounces)	34.00

Sources of Vitamin A (continued)

Food	Quantity	Percent of U.S. RDA
Cherries; red, sour, pitted (canned with water)	1 cup	33.20
Tomatoes, raw	1 medium	32.80
Spaghetti with meat balls, tomato sauce (homemade)	1 cup	31.80
Orange-apricot juice drink	1 cup	28.80
Finnan haddie	3 ounces	27.38
Peaches, raw	1 medium	26.40
Liverwurst, fresh	2 slices (¼-inch thick)	25.40
Milk, skim (fortified with vitamin A)	1 cup	10.00
Milk, whole	1 cup	6.20

Compiled from CONSUMER GUIDE® magazine Nutrition Data Bank.

Continued from page 71

sess known as chlorophyll. Americans get about half their vitamin A as retinol from animal sources and half as carotenes from plant sources. See the table on pages 72-75 for a list of good food sources of vitamin A and the percent of the U.S. RDA they provide.

Dietary Requirements for Vitamin A

The Recommended Dietary Allowance (RDA) for vitamin A is 1,000 retinol equivalents (RE) for men and 800 RE for women. Since one RE is equal to 5 IU,

Vitamin A: Retinol

the amounts listed are equivalent to 5,000 international units (IU) for men and 4,000 IU for women. Retinol equivalents are the preferred way for measuring vitamin A value because they take into account the fact that the vitamin is obtained in two forms, as retinol and also as carotene. International units are still used on labels however, because labeling regulations were formulated before REs were in use.

The RDAs of vitamin A for children can be found on the RDA table I, page 23. Because children are growing rapidly, they're at greater risk than adults of developing vitamin A deficiency and the eye problems it may cause.

It's not necessary to rigidly follow the RDA for vitamin A each day. Since vitamin A is not soluble in water, excess amounts of the vitamin do not leave the body in the urine. The excesses accumulate in the liver and can be tapped as a source whenever dietary intake of the vitamin is too low. For most adults it would take months to deplete this storage. As long as you have a well-balanced diet that includes milk, cheese, butter or margarine, and yellow and green vegetables, your overall intake should be sufficient to provide the amount of vitamin A that your body needs.

Your intake of vitamin A can be flexible from day to day. For example, eating liver or carrots on a given day may supply you with more than the recommended daily allowance for vitamin A. This, in turn, can help you make up for not meeting the RDA the day before. It's important to note, however, that if

Vitamin A: Retinol

most of the vitamin A in your diet comes from retinol in animal foods, you can get by with less than the RDA, but if you're a strict vegetarian and only get your supply of vitamin A from carotenes in vegetables, you will need a little more.

The table on pages 78-79 can help you identify the vitamin A content in two typical daily diets.

Deficiency of Vitamin A

An early warning sign of vitamin A deficiency is the inability to see well in the dark. As the condition progresses, the outer layers of the eyes become dry, thickened, and cloudy. Eventually, if left untreated, severe vitamin A deficiency causes blindness.

Vitamin A deficiency also causes the skin to become dry and rough, taking on a kind of "goose flesh" appearance. *Goose flesh* can be distinguished from *goose pimples* that result from exposure to cold temperatures, since the latter can be smoothed away by rubbing. In addition, deficiency of vitamin A increases susceptibility to infectious diseases, because the linings of the gastrointestinal and respiratory tracts are damaged and can't act effectively as barriers to keep bacteria from entering the body. Infections of the vagina are also more likely to occur when the body is vitamin A deficient.

To prevent deficiency, some developing countries have introduced programs to encourage people to

Continued on page 78

Vitamin A: Retinol

Vitamin A Content in Two Daily Diets

Typical Day's Diet for Woman (1,700 Calories)		IU of Vitamin A
Breakfast	4 ounces orange juice	270
	1 ounce enriched corn flakes	1,250
	1 slice enriched white toast	none
	1 pat butter	150
	1 cup 2-percent milk	500
	Black coffee	none
Lunch	Sandwich: 2 slices whole-wheat bread, 1 slice American cheese, 2 ounces boiled ham	490
	1 cup skim milk (fortified)	500
	½ cup cole slaw	60
Dinner	½ chicken breast, fried	70
	1 medium baked potato	none
	1 cup tossed green salad	180
	½ cup peas, cooked	480
	1 enriched dinner roll	none
	2 pats butter	300
	½ cup ice cream	270
	Black coffee	none
Total		**4,520**
RDA		**4,000**

Compiled from U.S.D.A. *Home and Garden Bulletin No. 72*, Washington, D.C., revised April 1977.

Continued from page 77
eat foods with high vitamin A value. Some countries fortify foods with vitamin A and/or provide large doses of the vitamin to children at six month intervals.

Vitamin A Content in Two Daily Diets

Typical Day's Diet for Teenage Boy (3,000 Calories)		IU of Vitamin A
Breakfast	½ medium pink grapefruit	540
	2 scrambled eggs	620
	2 slices enriched white toast	none
	1 pat butter	150
	1 cup whole milk	310
Lunch	1 cheeseburger	360
	2 cups whole milk	620
	10 large French-fried potatoes	none
	1 medium banana	230
Dinner	4 ounces round steak	25
	1 cup green beans	780
	1 cup mashed potatoes	40
	Lettuce and tomato salad	400
	2 slices enriched white bread	none
	1 pat butter	150
	1 cup whole milk	310
	4 chocolate chip cookies	50
Snacks	Cola drink	none
	½ cup ice cream	270
	¼ of 14-inch cheese pizza	200
Total		**5,055**
RDA		**5,000**

Compiled from U.S.D.A. *Home and Garden Bulletin, No. 72,* Washington, D.C., revised April 1977.

Vitamin A deficiency is common in the United States among low-income groups. Deficiency can also occur in people who eat very low fat diets or in those who

Vitamin A: Retinol

experience fat malabsorption due to conditions such as celiac disease or infectious hepatitis.

Mineral oil, when used as a lubricant to combat constipation, can cause a deficiency of vitamin A and other fat-soluble vitamins, since they dissolve in the oil and pass out of the body.

Vitamin A Use and Misuse

Children with xerophthalmia are given large doses of vitamin A at the start of treatment. After a few days, the dose is decreased.

Diseases such as obstructive jaundice or cystic fibrosis cause poor absorption of dietary fat and fat-soluble vitamins. People who have these diseases may have adequate amounts of vitamin A in their diets but still develop a deficiency because the disease reduces the amount of vitamin absorbed. To overcome this obstacle, doctors may prescribe water-soluble forms of vitamin A in amounts greater than the RDA.

A disease that is accompanied by prolonged fever, such as infectious hepatitis or rheumatic fever, may rapidly deplete the liver's reserves of vitamin A. As part of the treatment, vitamin A may be prescribed in amounts greater than the RDA to prevent deficiency.

Vitamin A derivatives are used to treat skin disorders. Accutane (13-cis retinoic acid) is an oral medication used for severe cystic acne. Because of the possibility of such serious side effects as liver damage and elevated blood triglycerides, treatment with this medication must be closely monitored by a doctor. Pregnant women should not use Accutane as it can cause serious birth defects and spontaneous abortion. A warning about the possible dangers for pregnant women appears on the product label.

Substances used topically have less potential for serious side effects than medications taken orally. Retin-A (all-trans-retinoic acid) is a topical medication for acne. It has been prescribed along with Minoxidil to treat baldness. This medication is also used to reduce wrinkles and reverse the effects of sun-damaged skin. Another vitamin A derivative, Etretinate, has been successfully used, in some cases, in the treatment of psoriasis.

Research has shown that people who have a high intake of beta-carotene, the form of carotene with the greatest vitamin A value, are less likely to develop lung cancer. Even among smokers, lung cancer is less likely to occur in those people who have high dietary levels of vegetables containing beta-carotene. Taking a vitamin A supplement in pill form does not appear to have the same effect. However, more research is needed to verify this.

Large amounts of vitamin A are toxic. One massive dose or large doses taken over an extended period of time can cause hair loss, joint pain, nausea, bone and muscle soreness, headaches, dry flaky skin, diarrhea, rashes, enlarged liver and spleen, cessation

Vitamin A: Retinol

of menstruation, and stunted growth. Excess carotenes accumulate in the blood and cause yellowing of the skin especially on the palms and soles of the feet. Too much carotene in the diet may be a factor in the amenorrhea (lack of menstrual periods) found in females who control their weight with large amounts of exercise coupled with diets emphasizing vegetables high in carotene. Carotene-containing tanning pills used in Europe have been reported to cause infertility in women.

Experts do not agree on how much vitamin A is too much, but toxic reactions have followed single doses of 500,000 IU in adults and 75,000 IU in children. Doses of only five to ten times the RDA for vitamin A can cause toxicity when taken over a long period of time.

The danger of toxicity may be compounded by "overage." This refers to the manufacturers' practice of including in supplements more than the labeled amount of some vitamins to ensure the vitamins' stated potency throughout its shelf life. For example, the overage may be as high as 40 percent for vitamin A. This means that a supplement with a labeled dose of 25,000 IU may actually provide as much as 35,000 IU. These additional amounts increase the risk of overdose.

In a few reported instances, vitamin A toxicity has occurred after eating large amounts of beef or chicken liver. Remember that vitamin A is stored in the liver, so that eating this organ meat daily may provide more of the vitamin than is desirable.

Vitamin D: Cholecalciferol

Fifty years ago, few children in tropical countries developed the malformed bones and teeth characteristic of rickets. Yet, many children in temperate climates and large industrial cities did. Why the difference from one region to another? The answer involves the "sunshine" vitamin—vitamin D.

The children in tropical countries were exposed to sunlight year-round. If you recall, skin contains a substance known as provitamin D that can be converted to vitamin D when exposed to sunlight. Since these children had ample opportunity for exposure, their skin could form adequate amounts of vitamin D and thus prevent the symptoms of rickets. Children in temperate zones, however, got little exposure to the sun during the winter months, and their skin could not make enough vitamin D. Neither could the skin of children in large, industrial cities, because the smoke-filled air filtered out much of the sun's ultraviolet light.

In recent years, cases of rickets are seldom seen in the United States. The incidence of rickets has been

Vitamin D: Cholecalciferol

cut dramatically by the increased availability of milk fortified with vitamin D. Milk was chosen in this country as the medium for fortification because children usually drink it in large quantity. Milk was also selected because it's the single best source of calcium in the American diet. What better place to add the vitamin that actually helps the body use its calcium supply?

Proof of the effectiveness of the vitamin D-fortification program is the virtual disappearance of rickets in the United States. Today when rickets is found, it can usually be traced to poverty, neglect, or ignorance.

History

In the early 1900s, rickets afflicted large numbers of children in this country. While searching for the cause of the disease, researchers fed various diets to experimental animals. Those diets that prevented calcium from depositing in the bones produced the soft bones that are characteristic of rickets. From this research, investigators concluded that rickets was actually a vitamin deficiency disease.

Yet, they became perplexed when they discovered that ultraviolet light also played a part in deficiency prevention. Nutritionists in the 1920s found that rickets could be prevented or cured by feeding children cod liver oil or food that had been exposed to ultraviolet light. Nutritionists also found that rickets could be prevented by exposing children to direct

Vitamin D: Cholecalciferol

sunlight or the light from a sunlamp. The explanation for these findings didn't come for several years.

Cod liver oil was found to be effective in the treatment of rickets because it contained vitamin D. Ultraviolet light was also effective because it changed a substance in plant foods, *ergosterol,* into a form of the vitamin called vitamin D_2. Ultraviolet light thus provided the essential nutrient in plant foods where none existed before. Direct sunlight and ultraviolet light from a sunlamp also provided vitamin D by transforming a substance found in the human skin into vitamin D_3.

Function of Vitamin D

Vitamin D is necessary to help the body absorb the minerals calcium and phosphorus for the growth and development of bones and teeth.

In addition to quantities of vitamin D acquired in the diet, a substance called provitamin D that's found in the skin can be converted to vitamin D in the presence of ultraviolet rays.

Whether derived from food or made in the skin, vitamin D first travels to the liver, where it undergoes a chemical change. In its new form, vitamin D moves through the bloodstream to the kidneys, where it undergoes another change to become the active form of the vitamin. This active form (dihydroxy vitamin D) assists the body in its absorption of calcium and phosphorus.

Vitamin D: Cholecalciferol

Sources of Vitamin D

There are few foods that naturally contain significant amounts of vitamin D. Butter, cream, egg yolk, and liver contain small amounts. Almost all milk of any type—whole, low-fat, skim, evaporated, or dry—is fortified with vitamin D at a level of 400 international units (IU) per quart. Some cereals and milk flavorings are also fortified with vitamin D.

Cod liver oil, as a supplement, contains 1,200 IUs of vitamin D per tablespoon.

It's been estimated that a fair-skinned person can make a sufficient quantity of vitamin D with only 30 minutes of sun exposure per day. It would take three hours for a dark-skinned person to make an equal amount of the vitamin because the pigment in the skin filters out the ultraviolet rays. Clouds, smog, clothing, and even window glass will do the same. Housebound people, therefore, and those with dark skin are more likely to be deficient in vitamin D.

With the recent emphasis on the use of sunscreens to protect the skin from the damaging effects of the sun, it may be more important to get sufficient amounts of this vitamin from foods.

Dietary Requirements for Vitamin D

Since 1980, vitamin D has been measured in micrograms (μg) as well as in international units (IU). The

Continued on page 88

Vitamin D: Cholecalciferol

Sources of Vitamin D

Food	Amount	IU	Percent of U.S. RDA
Product 19, Kellogg's	1 cup	200	50
Most, Kellogg's	1 cup	200	50
Dairy Queen Malt	large	140	35
Ovaltine	1 cup	139	35
Milk, fortified	1 cup	100	25
Skim milk, fortified	1 cup	100	25
Jack in the Box Breakfast Jack sandwich	1	51	13
McDonald's Egg McMuffin	1	46	11
Liver, beef, cooked	2½ ounces	46	11
Liver, pork, cooked	2½ ounces	46	11
McDonald's Chocolate shake	1	44	11
Special K, Kellogg's	1 cup	40	10
Crispix, Kellogg's	¾ cup	40	10
Kix, General Mills	1½ cups	40	10
ET Cereal, General Mills	1 cup	40	10
Milk Break, Milk Bar	1	40	10
McDonald's Big Mac	1	33	8
Egg	1 medium	27	7
Eggnog	½ cup	21	5
Chicken liver, cooked	2½ ounces	20	5
Liver, calves', cooked	2½ ounces	12	3
Butter	1 teaspoon	5	1
Cream, light	2 tablespoons	4	1

The RDA for vitamin D is 200 IU for adults. The U.S. RDA (labeling tool) for vitamin D is 400 IU.

Vitamin D: Cholecalciferol

Continued from page 86
Recommended Dietary Allowance (RDA) for children and women who are pregnant or breast-feeding is 10 μg (400 IU). For all other adults, the RDA is 5 μg (200 IU). One quart of fortified milk supplies 400 IU, 200 IU in a pint.

Deficiency of Vitamin D

In children, vitamin D deficiency causes rickets. One of its common signs is bowlegs. Another sign is bead-like swellings on the ribs, a condition known as rachitic rosary. Teething is usually late, and teeth are susceptible to decay. Rickets is only rarely seen in the United States today, but recently some cases have been reported in low-income black children, vegetarian children, and infants who were breast-fed for an extended period of time. These children appear to be particularly vulnerable.

The counterpart of rickets in adults is osteomalacia, loss of calcium and protein from the bones due to insufficient vitamin D. In developing countries, osteomalacia is prevalent in women who have low intakes of calcium and vitamin D, along with several closely spaced pregnancies that are followed by long periods of breast-feeding.

Use and Misuse of Vitamin D

Supplements of vitamin D should be taken by strict vegetarians who do not get enough sunlight. Breast-fed babies are routinely given vitamin D supplements. Formula-fed infants receive the recommended amount in commercial infant formula and do not require additional supplementation.

The standard treatment for rickets is a fairly high dose of vitamin D given under a doctor's supervision. The active form of the vitamin is sometimes used in those cases where normal conversion of vitamin D to the dihydroxy form is inadequate.

Vitamin D is the most toxic of all the vitamins. As little as 2,000 IU a day is the threshhold of toxicity for most children. Symptoms of overdose include diarrhea, nausea, headache, and elevated calcium levels in the blood (hypercalcemia). Hypercalcemia is very serious since it can lead to calcium deposits in the kidneys, heart, and other tissues, causing irreversible damage.

Because of the potential for harmful overdose, large amounts of vitamin D should not be taken. In the past, 50,000 IU (250 times the RDA for adults) was used as a treatment for arthritis. There was no proven benefit from this approach, and it's no longer recommended.

The claim is sometimes made that natural sources of vitamin D like cod liver oil are not toxic. This is not true; toxic symptoms have developed in children who were given large doses of cod liver oil. Supplements, whether natural or synthetic, should not be taken in amounts that supply more than the RDA for the vitamins.

Vitamin E: Tocopherol

If ever a vitamin has received more credit than it deserves, that's vitamin E. Retail sales of vitamin E supplements have soared. Yet, there's no scientific evidence to back the claims that megadoses can promote physical endurance, enhance sexual potency, prevent heart attacks, slow the aging process, smooth scars, lower blood fat levels, reverse heart attack damage, aid hot flashes and other menopausal symptoms, or produce any of the other minor miracles attributed to it. Millions of consumers—despite scientific information to the contrary—remain devoted to vitamin E and refuse to replace faith and the fiction of false publicity with fact.

What exactly is vitamin E? What can it do? And how did it gain its reputation as a miracle worker?

History

The first indication for the existence of vitamin E came in 1922. Laboratory rats fed purified diets lost their reproductive ability; male rats became sterile, and female rats reabsorbed their fetuses or delivered deformed or stillborn offspring. When foods such as lettuce, wheat, meat, or butter were added to the animals' diets, an unknown factor was supplied which prevented these reproductive problems. Isolated in 1936, the factor was named *tocopherol* from the Greek, meaning "to bring forth offspring." Later, the substance became known as vitamin E.

It was discovered that vitamin E is not a single compound, but several different compounds, all with vitamin E activity. One, known as alpha-tocopherol, has the greatest activity. (Its derivative, alpha-tocopherol acetate, is commonly used in commercial supplements.) Other compounds with vitamin E activity are beta-tocopherol, gamma-tocopherol and delta-tocopherol.

Following the discovery of vitamin E, deficiency studies were conducted using various animal species. It soon became obvious that deficiency symptoms varied from one species to another. In rabbits, a degenerative muscle disease was the result of vitamin E deficiency, and the symptoms were corrected by the addition of the vitamin to the animals' diets. Because these symptoms were similar to those seen in human subjects with muscular dystrophy, researchers hoped that this crippling disease in humans could be cured or prevented with vitamin E. It was hoped, too, that the vitamin might be helpful in human cases of infertility and sterility. However, studies in humans since 1938 have failed to show any such benefits.

Vitamin E: Tocopherol

Here lies the foundation for some of the false claims that have surrounded vitamin E as an aid for sexual potency and muscle disorders. Additional claims have accumulated over the years.

Function of Vitamin E

Vitamin E functions as an antioxidant in the cells and tissues of the body. It helps to prevent undesirable oxidation reactions by inhibiting the combination of body substances with oxygen. It does this by combining with the oxygen itself. Because of this, it protects polyunsaturated fats and other oxygen-sensitive compounds like vitamin A from being destroyed. Its antioxidant function is important to cell membranes. For example, vitamin E protects lung cells that are in constant contact with oxygen and white cells that help the body fight disease. A deficiency of this vitamin suppresses the immune system and renders the body susceptible to infection.

Vitamin E also acts as an antioxidant in foods. The vitamin E in vegetable oils helps to keep them from being oxidized and becoming rancid. This property makes vitamin E a useful food additive as a preservative.

Sources of Vitamin E

Corn, cottonseed, soybean, safflower, and wheat germ oil, and margarines made from these oils are all good sources of vitamin E. Fruits, vegetables, and whole grains have smaller amounts. Refining grains reduces their vitamin E content, as does commercial processing and storage of food. Fresh and lightly processed foods are the best sources. Because it's found in so many foods, eating a well-balanced, varied diet should ensure an ample supply of vitamin E.

Dietary Requirements for Vitamin E

The Recommended Dietary Allowance (RDA) for vitamin E is 10 mg of D-alpha-tocopherol. This amount is equal to 15 IU. One mg of D-alpha-tocopherol is equal to 1.5 IU.

Deficiency of Vitamin E

Because vitamin E is found in so many foods, and because the average person has a supply of the vitamin stored in his or her fat deposits, it's not common to find a deficiency in people on normal diets.

Mild deficiency may be seen when intestinal absorption is reduced as may occur in diseases of the liver, gall bladder, or pancreas. In this situation, a vitamin supplement is useful. A very low-fat diet, high in processed foods, might cause a deficiency because vitamin E is destroyed by extensive heating at high temperatures.

At one time, vitamin E supplements were recommended for people with high polyunsaturated fat

Continued on page 95

Vitamin E: Tocopherol

Sources of Vitamin E

Food	Amount	IU	Percent of U.S. RDA
Total	1 cup	30.0	100
Most, Kellogg's	1 cup	30.0	100
Wheat germ oil	1 tablespoon	28.3	93
Walnut oil	1 tablespoon	13.1	43
Sunflower oil	1 tablespoon	10.3	30
Sweet potato	1 medium	9.7	30
Cottonseed oil	1 tablespoon	8.9	30
Safflower oil	1 tablespoon	8.5	28
Walnuts	11 halves	4.6	17
Asparagus	5-6 spears	3.7	13
Corn oil	1 tablespoon	3.6	13
Sunflower seeds	2 tablespoons	3.5	13
Soybean oil	1 tablespoon	3.4	13
Almonds	7 nuts	3.0	10
Hazelnuts	5 nuts	2.4	8
Brussels sprouts	3 large	2.3	8
Broccoli	1 cup	2.2	8
Wheat germ	2 tablespoons	2.1	6
Apple	1 medium	1.8	6
Beans, dry	½ cup	1.6	5
Corn	1 ear	1.5	5
Whole-wheat flour	⅓ cup	1.5	5
Parsnip	½ large	1.5	5
Brazil nuts	4 nuts	1.4	5
Peanuts	1 tablespoon	1.4	5
Pear	1 medium	1.2	4
Brown rice, uncooked	⅓ cup	1.1	4

Sources of Vitamin E (continued)

Food	Amount	IU	Percent of U.S. RDA
Banana	1 medium	.7	2
Carrot	1 medium	.6	2
Egg	1 large	.6	2
Grapefruit	½ medium	.6	2
Plum	1 large	.6	2
Butter	1 tablespoon	.5	2
Tomato	1 medium	.5	2
Raspberries	½ cup	.4	1
Cornmeal, uncooked	¼ cup	.4	1
Oatmeal, uncooked	¼ cup	.4	1
Orange	1 medium	.4	1

The RDA for vitamin E is 15 IU for males, 12 IU for females. The U.S. RDA (labeling tool) for vitamin E is 30 IU.

Continued from page 93

intakes. Experts now feel this isn't necessary since the polyunsaturated fats themselves are good sources of vitamin E.

Vitamin E deficiency in newborn babies, especially those born prematurely, may occur because there's little transfer of the vitamin from the mother to the developing fetus until the last weeks of pregnancy. The deficiency may result in hemolytic anemia, a condition in which the red blood cells are fragile and rupture (hemolyze) at an unusually rapid rate. With administration of vitamin E supplements, the problem can be cured.

Vitamin E: Tocopherol

Vitamin E Use and Misuse

Vitamin E may be useful to reduce or prevent oxygen damage to the retina of premature babies. Vitamin E therapy may also be useful to treat pains in the calf muscles that occur at night or during exercise. Another more controversial use of vitamin E supplements is for the treatment of painful, benign breast lumps (fibrocystic breast disease). Caffeine reduction is often used along with vitamin E to treat this condition.

Ongoing animal studies suggest that vitamin E may be useful in reducing lung damage caused by air pollution. Common air pollutants like ozone and nitrogen dioxide may cause lung damage. It appears that their activity can be reduced by vitamin E.

Vitamin E applied to cuts may increase the healing rate since it minimizes oxidation reactions in the wound. The value of vitamin E in reducing the formation of stretch marks that occur in pregnancy has been claimed in many anecdotal reports, but it has not yet been proven scientifically.

Vitamin E deficiency in animals causes fertility problems and muscle degeneration. Unfortunately, research shows that vitamin E does not have a role in similar problems in humans.

While vitamin E can slow down the oxidation of fats in body cells that occurs in aging, it hasn't been shown to increase lifespan in animals. Neither has it been shown to control signs of aging such as wrinkling skin or graying hair.

Many women report that vitamin E has helped reduce hot flashes and other symptoms of menopause. These are considered anecdotal reports and do not stand up to scientific scrutiny.

Vitamin E seems to be fairly safe when taken in amounts of 400 IUs daily for a long time. Excess vitamin E, however, taken in amounts larger than this, may prolong blood clotting. Megadoses should not be taken by people on anticoagulant therapy (blood thinners) as they may substantially increase blood-clotting time.

Vitamin K: Naphthoquinone

The "k" in vitamin K was derived from the Danish word "koagulation," meaning "blood clotting," and is used as the vitamin's designation because it precisely reflects its function in the human body.

History

The importance of a dietary factor in blood clotting was first recognized by Danish scientist Henrik Dam. In 1929, he reported that chicks who were fed diets lacking a particular dietary factor experienced hemorrhages because their blood was slow to form the clots needed to control bleeding. The dietary factor, then called the "antihemorrhagic factor," turned out to be vitamin K.

Function of Vitamin K

Vitamin K is needed to make proteins used in blood clotting. When there's a deficiency of the vitamin,

Vitamin K: Naphthoquinone

the amount of time it takes for blood to clot increases. Consequently, the amount of blood lost increases as well. Vitamin K also works along with vitamin D to make a protein that helps regulate blood calcium levels. Calcium is another factor that's necessary for the clotting process to occur.

Sources of Vitamin K

The best sources of vitamin K are green, leafy vegetables like cabbage, turnip greens, broccoli, lettuce, and spinach. Beef liver is another good source, while chicken liver, pork liver, milk, and eggs contain less of the vitamin.

Bacteria living in the human digestive tract produce vitamin K. For us, that represents another important source of the vitamin. It's estimated that we get half of the vitamin K we use from food, and the other half from the bacteria in our intestines.

Dietary Requirements for Vitamin K

Because less information is known about vitamin K than some of the other vitamins, an *estimated safe and adequate range of intake* is given in the RDA tables *rather than a recommendation*. The suggested range of intake is 70 to 140 µg. A typical well-balanced diet in the United States has been found to supply 300 to 500 µg of vitamin K. This is more than enough to meet average dietary needs.

Continued on page 101

Vitamin K: Naphthoquinone

Sources of Vitamin K*

Food	Amount	Micrograms
Turnip greens, cooked	⅔ cup	650
Lettuce	¼ head	129
Cabbage, cooked	⅔ cup	125
Liver, beef	3 ounces	110
Broccoli, cooked	½ cup	100
Spinach, cooked	½ cup	80
Asparagus, cooked	⅔ cup	57
Liver, pork	3 ounces	30
Peas, cooked	⅔ cup	19
Ham	3 ounces	18
Green beans, cooked	¾ cup	14
Cheese	1 ounce	14
Egg	1	11
Ground beef, raw	4 ounces	10.5
Milk	1 cup	10
Liver, chicken	3 ounces	8
Peach	1 medium	8
Butter	1 tablespoon	6
Tomato	1 small	5
Banana	1 medium	3
Applesauce	⅓ cup	2
Corn oil	1 tablespoon	2
Bread	1 slice	1

The RDA for vitamin K is 70-140 µg. *There is no nutrition labeling recommendation for vitamin K.

*This nutrient is not found in the main table of the RDA because there is less information known about it; therefore, a *range of estimated safe and adequate daily dietary intake* is suggested rather than a specific recommendation.

Vitamin K: Naphthoquinone

Continued from page 99
Deficiency of Vitamin K

As we've said, a deficiency of vitamin K due to a lack of the vitamin in our dietary intake isn't a likely possibility. However, liver or gall bladder disease, or any disease of the intestinal tract that interferes with absorption of fats and fat-soluble vitamins may cause a deficiency. Long-term use of oral antibiotics kills off the bacteria in the intestines that manufacture the vitamin. This regimen may lead to a deficiency, especially if coupled with the use of a formula diet that doesn't contain vitamin K.

Use of mineral oil, or use of some of the medications that are prescribed to lower cholesterol in the blood, such as cholestyramine, interferes with the absorption of vitamin K and the other fat-soluble vitamins. Over extended periods of time, this, too, may lead to deficiency.

Newborn babies, especially those born prematurely, are born with little vitamin K. In addition, for the first couple of days after birth, the baby's intestinal tract has no bacteria to make the vitamin. Because the lack of vitamin K could lead to bleeding problems, babies are routinely given a supplement of vitamin K soon after birth.

Vitamin K Use and Misuse

Vitamin K supplements are given to people who can-

Vitamin K: Naphthoquinone

not absorb the vitamin normally or sometimes to people on long-term antibiotic therapy. Vitamin K may be given before surgery, but is only of value in this situation if there's a deficiency.

Anticoagulants (blood thinners, such as dicoumarol) are used in the treatment of heart disease and other diseases that cause the blood to clot too easily. Blood thinners interfere with the action of vitamin K and slow down the clotting process. People taking anti-coagulants may reduce this action of the drug by increasing their intake of vitamin K-rich foods.

Large doses of vitamin K have been reported to cause bleeding. Water-soluble forms of vitamin K have occasionally caused toxicity (red cell breakdown, jaundice, and brain damage) when given to infants or pregnant women.

Vitamin B$_1$: Thiamin

The discovery of thiamin in the 1930s was the key that unlocked the mystery of a disease—a disease born of technology.

Beriberi, a debilitating and often fatal ailment, didn't become a serious health problem among the rice-eating peoples of the Orient until the end of the 19th century. At that time, mills began to polish rice—a process that would remove the outer brown layers of the grain and leave behind smooth white kernels. When the rice was stripped of its bran, it lost much of the thiamin it contained. People who ate the polished rice were deprived of this vitamin, and the incidence of beriberi rose to an epidemic level. A similar situation arose in countries where wheat was a staple food, and refined white flour began to replace that of whole wheat.

Before mills made refined grains available to many people, beriberi was uncommon. With the rise of commercial milling of rice and other cereals came a swift increase in the incidence of the disease. The increased prevalence spurred efforts to find its cause and cure. Still, the search took almost 50 years and didn't end until the vitamin thiamin was discovered.

History

K. Takaki, a medical officer in the Japanese navy, was the first to suspect that diet had a bearing on beriberi. In the 1880s, Takaki sought the root of this disease, which afflicted large numbers of Japanese sailors on long voyages. The disease was so rampant that on one nine-month voyage, 169 of the 276 crew members aboard one ship developed beriberi, and 25 of them died. To test his belief that diet was at fault, Takaki added meat and milk to the rice diet of the sailors. He found that during a similar voyage, only a few men came down with the malady—only those men who refused to eat the milk and meat.

Further evidence of the relationship between diet and beriberi came from Java, where the Dutch physician Cristiaan Eijkman found that chickens who were fed polished rice exhibited symptoms similar to those of beriberi. When he fed the chickens unpolished rice, the symptoms disappeared. Eijkman extended his experiments to humans and confirmed that beriberi could be prevented or cured if unpolished rice were substituted for polished grain.

The explanation for these findings wasn't provided until 1901, when Gerrit Grijns, a nutrition researcher also working in Java, suggested that unpolished rice contained an unknown substance that prevented

Vitamin B₁: Thiamin

beriberi. In 1910, chemist Robert Williams began a similar search. While working in the Philippines, he was asked by a member of the U.S. Army Medical Corps to analyze a brown liquid that had been extracted from rice polishings. Williams painstakingly tested the substances from the liquid for their effect on polyneuritis, a disease among chickens that is similar to beriberi. It was 1934 before Williams isolated the substance that would solve the mystery of beriberi. It was the vitamin thiamin.

Function of Thiamin

Like other B-complex vitamins, thiamin acts as a biologic catalyst, or coenzyme. As a coenzyme, thiamin participates in the long chain of reactions that provides energy for the body to function, and heat for the body to maintain a constant temperature. Thiamin is also involved in the synthesis of fats and in protein metabolism. In addition, thiamin is needed for normal functioning of the nervous system.

Sources of Thiamin

The term "enriched" seen on food labels means that three "B" vitamins—thiamin, niacin, and riboflavin—plus one mineral, iron, have been added to that food. That's why when you eat enriched breads and cereals they're as good a source of thiamin as natural sources, like whole grains. Pork is an especially rich source of the vitamin. Ham, oysters, green peas, and

Continued on page 107

Vitamin B$_1$: Thiamin

Sources of Thiamin

Food	Quantity	Percent of U.S. RDA
Pistachio nuts	1 cup	62.67
Pecan halves	1 cup	62.00
Pork roast	3 ounces	52.00
Oatmeal, ready-to-serve	¾ cup	50.73
Filberts or hazelnuts	1 cup	42.67
Cashews, roasted	1 cup	40.00
Macadamia nuts	1 cup	32.00
Peas; green, cooked	1 cup	29.33
Ham, roasted	3 ounces	26.67
Dry beans, peas; cooked	1 cup	16.67
Peanuts	½ cup	15.33
Rice; enriched, cooked	1 cup	15.33
Beef liver	3 ounces	14.67
Orange juice	1 cup	14.67
Bread, white enriched	2 slices	13.33
Macaroni; cooked, enriched	1 cup	13.33
Orange	1 medium	8.67
Bread, whole-wheat	2 slices	8.00
Potato, baked	1 medium	6.67
Milk, whole or skim	1 cup	6.00
Frankfurter	1	5.33
Yogurt	1 cup	5.33
Ground beef	3 ounces	4.67
Cottage cheese	1 cup	3.33
Chicken	3 ounces	2.67
Fish	3 ounces	2.00-4.00

Vitamin B$_1$: Thiamin

Continued from page 105

lima beans are also good sources. In most other foods, thiamin is found in only very small amounts. Other thiamin sources are listed on page 106.

Thiamin is not very stable and can be easily destroyed by high cooking temperatures. As a water-soluble vitamin, it also leaches out from food into the cooking water. In order to preserve the thiamin values of foods, they should be cooked at low temperatures in small amounts of water for the shortest time possible. Steaming and microwaving are good cooking choices for preserving vitamin values.

Some people add baking soda to their vegetables to help preserve their bright green color during cooking. But the baking soda makes the vegetables lose their shape and consistency, as well as destroying the thiamin content. Sulfites, used as preservatives, also destroy thiamin.

Dietary Requirements for Thiamin

The Recommended Dietary Allowance (RDA) for thiamin is related to the amount of calories taken in. For every 1,000 calories, 0.5 mg of thiamin is needed. Thiamin intake should be at least 1.0 mg per day, even if the total calorie intake is less than 2,000.

The RDA is 1.4 mg of thiamin for men and 1.0 mg for women. During pregnancy or nursing, when

Continued on page 109

Vitamin B$_1$: Thiamin

Thiamin Content
of Common Foods

Food	Quantity	Milligrams of Thiamin
Milk–Dairy Group		
Milk, whole or skim	1 cup	0.09
Yogurt	1 cup	0.08
Cottage cheese	1 cup	0.05
Ice cream	1 cup	0.05
Meat–Protein Group		
Pork roast	3 ounces	0.78
Pork chop, cooked	1	0.63
Ham	3 ounces	0.40
Dry beans, peas; cooked	1 cup	0.25
Peanuts	½ cup	0.23
Beef liver	3 ounces	0.22
Bologna	2 slices	0.10
Frankfurter	1	0.08
Ground beef	3 ounces	0.07
Roast beef	3 ounces	0.05
Chicken	3 ounces	0.04
Fish	3 ounces	0.03 to 0.06
Fruits–Vegetables Group		
Peas, cooked	½ cup	0.22
Orange	1 medium	0.13
Asparagus	½ cup	0.11
Orange juice	4 ounces	0.11
Potatoes		
Baked	1 medium	0.10
French fries	10 pieces	0.07
Chips	10 pieces	0.04
Iceberg lettuce	¼ head	0.08

Thiamin Content
of Common Foods (continued)

Food	Quantity	Milligrams of Thiamin
Banana	1 medium	0.06
Cabbage, raw	1 cup	0.05
Green or snap beans	½ cup	0.05
Apple	1 medium	0.04
Carrot, raw	1 medium	0.04

Bread—Cereal/Grain Group

Food	Quantity	Milligrams of Thiamin
Ready-to-eat breakfast cereals (enriched)		
Total, Product 19	1 ounce each	1.50
King Vitaman	1 ounce	0.90
Wheaties, corn flakes, Bran Flakes	1 ounce each	0.37
Rice; enriched, cooked	1 cup	0.23
Macaroni, noodles, spaghetti; cooked (enriched)	1 cup	0.20
Bread, white enriched	1 slice	0.10
Bread, whole-wheat	1 slice	0.06

Compiled from product labels and U.S.D.A. *Home and Garden Bulletin No 72*, Washington, D.C., revised April 1977.

Continued from page 107

more calories are needed, there's an increased need for thiamin as well. A varied, well-balanced diet should easily supply the amount needed. The table on pages 108-109 shows the amount of thiamin supplied in common foods.

Vitamin B$_1$: Thiamin

Deficiency of Thiamin

In an East Indian dialect, beriberi means weakness, a chief symptom of one form of the disease—dry beriberi. Dry beriberi is characterized by numbness, muscle weakness, loss of appetite, and disorders of the nervous system. In contrast, wet beriberi is characterized by accumulation of water, especially in the legs. This severe form of the disease interferes with normal functioning of the heart and circulatory system, and may eventually cause heart failure.

Severe thiamin deficiency seldom occurs today in the Western world. However, alcoholics who eat little or no food for extended periods of time are susceptible to thiamin deficiency and may develop a pattern of neurologic symptoms known as Wernike-Korsakoff syndrome. Deficiency may also occur in people who make poor food choices through ignorance, neglect, or poverty. Usually diets that are deficient in thiamin are deficient in other B vitamins as well.

Thiamin Use and Misuse

Doses of 2 to 5 times the RDA level of thiamin are used to treat deficiency. Large doses are found in "anti-stress" supplements recommended by some to reduce stress and fatigue. Thiamin does not provide instant energy. It merely plays a part in the reactions that supply the body with energy. This vitamin has no known effect on fatigue unless it is caused by a thiamin deficiency. Large amounts of thiamin have not been shown to be toxic.

Vitamin B$_2$: Riboflavin

Riboflavin's story is a colorful one—it's yellow in fact. In the 1920s and 1930s, nutritionists were searching for a growth-promoting factor in food and, in their search, kept finding yellow substances. Meanwhile, biochemists were busy trying to solve some of the mysteries of metabolism and, in their efforts, kept running into a yellow enzyme. The yellow substances in the food and in part of the enzyme were both riboflavin.

History

Most nutritionists in the 1920s believed that there were only two unidentified essential nutrients, a fat-soluble "A" and a water-soluble "B." Soon, however, they found that there was a second water-soluble B compound, and they set to the task of identifying it.

During the course of their work, nutritionists gradually isolated growth-producing substances from liver,

Vitamin B$_2$: Riboflavin

eggs, milk, and grass. As you may have guessed, all of the substances were yellow. In 1933, L.E. Booher reported that she had also obtained a yellow, growth-promoting substance from milk whey. In addition, she observed that the darker the color of the substance, the greater its potency. Booher's observation was a clue that led nutritionists to the discovery that all the yellow growth-producing substances they had found in foods were one and the same: the water-soluble compound riboflavin.

While nutritionists were zeroing in on the yellow substance in food, biochemists were studying a yellow enzyme that was essential for the body's energy needs. The biochemists were eventually able to separate the enzyme into two parts: a colorless protein and a yellow organic compound. The yellow compound was riboflavin. The convergence of the lines of research provided an explanation for the growth-promoting properties of riboflavin and furnished information about its biochemical mechanism. This was the first indication to scientists that many of the B vitamins function as coenzymes.

Function of Riboflavin

Riboflavin doesn't act alone in the body. It works in concert with its B-complex kin. Along with other B vitamins, riboflavin acts as a coenzyme—the nonprotein, active portion of an enzyme—helping to metabolize carbohydrates, fats, and proteins. Riboflavin also has a role in the metabolism of other vitamins.

Vitamin B$_2$: Riboflavin

Sources of Riboflavin

Milk is the best source of riboflavin in the American diet. A glass of milk provides 1/4 of the Recommended Dietary Allowance for riboflavin for a man and 1/3 of the RDA for a woman. Other dairy products such as cheese, yogurt, and ice cream are also good sources of the vitamin. Meats, especially liver and kidney, and some green, leafy vegetables are other rich sources. Enriched breads and cereals have riboflavin added. See the table on pages 114-115 for a list of food sources of this vitamin.

Riboflavin is not easily destroyed by heat and oxygen, but it can be destroyed by light. It's estimated that milk can lose 1/2 or more of its riboflavin when exposed to sunlight for four to six hours. To prevent this from occurring, it's important not to store milk in clear glass or translucent plastic containers that may be exposed to light.

Dietary Requirements for Riboflavin

The Recommended Dietary Allowance (RDA) for riboflavin is 0.6 mg for every 1,000 calories taken in. This works out to be 1.6 mg each day for the average adult male and 1.2 mg for the average female. An additional 0.3 mg is recommended during pregnancy, and an additional 0.5 mg is suggested for women who are nursing. See the RDA table on page 24 for the amounts of riboflavin recommended for infants and children. The table on pages 117-118

Continued on page 116

Vitamin B$_2$: Riboflavin

Sources of Riboflavin

Food	Quantity	Percent of U.S. RDA
Beef liver	3 ounces	209.41
Almonds; whole, shelled	1 cup	77.06
Milk shake, thick (made from mix)	10 ounces	38.24
Roe, baked or broiled	3 ounces	38.24
Avocado, raw (late summer, fall: Florida)	1 whole	35.88
Buttermilk, from skim milk	1 cup	25.88
Avocado, raw (mid-late winter: California)	1 whole	25.29
Buttermilk, from whole milk	1 cup	24.12
Milk, whole or skim	1 cup	22.35
Cottage cheese	1 cup	20.00
Ice cream	1 cup	19.41
Yogurt (various types and flavors)	1 cup	18.82-31.17
Broccoli, cooked	1 cup	17.65
Spinach, cooked	1 cup	15.29
Asparagus, cooked	1 cup	12.94
Collards; leaves and stems, cooked	½ cup	11.76

Sources of Riboflavin (continued)

Food	Quantity	Percent of U.S. RDA
Peanuts	1 cup	11.76
Tuna	3 ounces	11.76
Pork chop, cooked	3½ ounces	11.18
Dandelion greens, cooked	½ cup	9.41
Beet greens, cooked	½ cup	8.82
Chicken	3 ounces	8.82
Egg	1 whole	8.82
Ground beef, cooked	3 ounces	8.82
Ham	3 ounces	8.82
Roast beef	3 ounces	8.82
Peas and beans; dried, cooked	1 cup	7.65
Cheese, natural and processed	1 ounce	6.47
Frankfurter	1	6.47
Brussels sprouts; frozen, cooked	3½ ounces	5.88
Green or snap beans	1 cup	5.88

Vitamin B$_2$: Riboflavin

Continued from page 113
shows the riboflavin content in common foods.

Deficiency of Riboflavin

When there's a deficiency of riboflavin, the skin becomes greasy, scaly, and dry. There may be cracks or fissures at the corners of the mouth (angular stomatitis), inflammation and soreness of the lips (cheilosis), and a smooth, reddish-purple tongue (glossitis).

Because prolonged deficiency of riboflavin causes severe eye damage in animals, it was supposed that some eye problems in people could be due to a lack of this vitamin. It's been suggested that cataracts might be due to a riboflavin deficiency, but there's little data to support this idea. Eye-related problems including hypersensitivity to light are noted as signs of riboflavin deficiency, but are most likely due to a deficiency of several of the "B" vitamins. Since the B vitamins work together in a sequence of reactions, a deficiency of one vitamin can effect the entire sequence.

Riboflavin Use and Misuse

Doses of as much as two to five times the RDA of riboflavin are used to treat deficiency. Therapeutic doses of riboflavin have not been shown to be beneficial in the treatment of any other condition.

Continued on page 119

Riboflavin Content
of Common Foods

Food	Quantity	Milligrams of Riboflavin
Milk—Dairy Group		
Milk shake, thick (made from mix)	10 ounces	0.65
Milk, whole or skim	1 cup	0.38
Cottage cheese	1 cup	0.34
Ice cream, ice milk	1 cup	0.33
Yogurt (various types and flavors)	1 cup	0.32-0.53
Cheese, natural and processed	1 ounce	0.11
Bread—Cereal/Grain Group		
Ready-to-eat breakfast cereals (enriched)	1 ounce	0.4-1.7
Macaroni; enriched, cooked	1 cup	0.12
Bread, white enriched	1 slice	0.06
Oatmeal, cooked	1 cup	0.05
Bread, whole wheat	1 slice	0.03
Rice, cooked	1 cup	0.02
Meat—Protein Group		
Beef liver	3 ounces	3.56
Ground beef	1 hamburger	0.20
Pork chop, cooked	1	0.18
Chicken	3 ounces	0.15
Egg	1 whole	0.15

Continued on next page

Vitamin B$_2$: Riboflavin

Riboflavin Content
of Common Foods (continued)

Food	Quantity	Milligrams of Riboflavin
Meat—Protein Group		
Ham	3 ounces	0.15
Roast beef	3 ounces	0.15
Peas and beans, cooked	1 cup	0.13
Bologna	2 slices	0.12
Frankfurter	1	0.11
Peanuts	½ cup	0.10
Tuna	3 ounces	0.10
Fruits—Vegetables Group		
Broccoli, cooked	½ cup	0.15
Spinach, cooked	½ cup	0.13
Squash, winter; baked	½ cup	0.13
Asparagus, cooked	½ cup	0.11
Banana	1 medium	0.07
Potato, baked	1 medium	0.07
Apple	1 medium	0.06
Green or snap beans	½ cup	0.05
Orange	1 medium	0.05
Strawberries, raw	½ cup	0.05
Carrot, raw	1 medium	0.02

Compiled from product labels and U.S.D.A. *Home and Garden Bulletin No. 72,* Washington, D.C., revised April 1977.

Vitamin B$_2$: Riboflavin

Continued from page 116

Large doses of riboflavin have not been reported to cause toxicity or any adverse reactions. However, large doses will cause the urine to appear bright yellow. This may cause some concern if the user is not aware of this possibility.

Niacin

What do heart disease and schizophrenia have in common? The need for supplements containing large amounts of the B-complex vitamin known as niacin, some people say. However, when psychiatrists and experts in heart disease looked past these claims and searched for sound scientific evidence, they discovered that in practice, and even in theory, *large doses of the vitamin are unwarranted*. Given in moderate doses, niacin *will* benefit a particular disease—the disease that led investigators along the road to the discovery of this vitamin.

History

The search for niacin, like that of other vitamins, was prompted by the quest for a cure for a specific disease. And like the search for other vitamins, the path that researchers followed took several wrong turns along the way.

In the early part of the 18th century, a disease characterized by red, rough skin began to appear in Europe. Almost 200 years later, the disease was still a scourge—at least for people in the southern United

States. The disease known as pellagra occurred in almost epidemic proportions in the South during the early 1900s. It appeared so often that many believed it was an infectious disease that spread from person to person. Others thought it was caused by eating spoiled corn. Still others felt that it was spread by a type of fly, because outbreaks of the malady were more severe in the spring during flies' hatching season.

Although pellagra *was* associated with corn-based diets, acceptance of the theory that it was caused by a dietary deficiency was slow in coming. One of the theory's first proponents, Dr. Joseph Goldberger, was convinced that the illness was caused by malnutrition. He began to experiment with the diets of children in a Mississippi orphanage who suffered from pellagra. After adding meat, milk, and eggs to their diets, he observed that the symptoms of the disease disappeared.

Then, in 1915, he conducted what has come to be considered a classic experiment in human nutrition. For six months, Goldberger ordered all the food that 11 volunteers from a Mississippi prison farm would eat. He selected foods that were prevalent in areas hard hit by pellagra. When Goldberger changed their diets to include lean meat, milk, or yeast, the symptoms vanished. The experiment provided solid proof that pellagra was the result of a dietary deficiency.

Yet, some physicians were still not completely convinced. Many remained skeptical until 1937, when

Niacin

Conrad Elvehjem and his co-workers at the University of Wisconsin reported that dogs with pellagra-like symptoms could be cured with a form of niacin called nicotinic acid. Soon, other investigators used nicotinic acid to cure pellagra in humans. And so it was. The mystery of pellagra had been solved.

Function of Niacin

Niacin occurs in two forms—nicotinic acid and nicotinamide. Both forms are found in foods. Nicotinic acid changes to nicotinamide in the body. Like the other B vitamins, niacin acts as a coenzyme in the metabolism of proteins, carbohydrates and fats.

Sources of Niacin

Niacin value in foods occurs as niacin itself (called preformed niacin), and also as the amino acid tryptophan, which can be converted to niacin in the body. In food composition tables, only the preformed niacin is listed, not the amount of niacin that could be made from tryptophan. Tryptophan, found in most proteins, is used primarily to build body tissue. It takes 60 mg of tryptophan to make 1 mg of niacin. *Niacin equivalent* is the term used to refer to either 1 mg of niacin or to 60 mg of tryptophan. It's estimated that in the average American diet, the amino acid tryptophan provides about 60 percent of the required amount of niacin. If a diet is adequate in

Continued on page 124

Sources of Niacin

Food	Quantity	Percent of U.S. RDA
Peanut halves; roasted, salted	1 cup	123.50
Product 19 breakfast cereal	1 ounce	100.00
Total breakfast cereal	1 ounce	100.00
Beef liver	3 ounces	70.00
Tuna; canned in water (solids and liquid)	3½ ounces	66.50
Turkey, roasted	3½ ounces	49.00
Chicken liver, cooked	2 ounces	47.00
Chicken, roasted	3½ ounces	45.00
Salmon, broiled or baked	3 ounces	41.50
Beef round; bottom, broiled	4 ounces	32.50
Lamb chop, cooked	3½ ounces	32.50
Chicken; canned, boned	3½ ounces	27.50
Pork chop, cooked	3½ ounces	27.50
Ground beef	3 ounces	23.00
Roast beef	3 ounces	22.50
Ham, baked	3 ounces	15.50
Peanut butter	1 tablespoon	12.00
Frankfurter; all-beef, cooked	1	7.00
Dried peas, beans; cooked	1 cup	6.50
Cottage cheese, creamed	1 cup	1.50
Yogurt	1 cup	1.50
Cheese, natural and processed	1 ounce	*
Egg	1 whole	*

*This food contains only a trace of pre-formed niacin. The food's tryptophan content gives it value as a source of the vitamin.

Compiled from CONSUMER GUIDE® magazine Nutrition Data Bank.

Niacin

Continued from page 122

protein, it will supply enough niacin equivalents to meet the daily need. The best sources of niacin or niacin equivalents, are foods that have a high protein content, such as meat, eggs, and peanuts. Other good sources of niacin, such as milk, actually provide more tryptophan than niacin. Mushrooms and greens are good vegetable sources. Niacin has also been added to enriched breads and cereals.

Dietary Requirements for Niacin

The RDA takes into account both the preformed niacin and that available from tryptophan. Together these make up the recommendation of 6.6 mg of niacin for each 1,000 calories taken in. For women, this should total no less than 13 mg (niacin equivalents) and for men, no less than 18 mg (niacin equivalents).

Deficiency of Niacin

The classic niacin deficiency disease is pellagra. At first, pellagra causes weakness, loss of appetite, and some digestive disturbances. As the disease progresses, the skin becomes rough and red in areas exposed to sunlight, heat, or irritation. Later, ulcers (open sores), diarrhea, dementia, or delirium develop. And finally, death may result if the condition is left untreated.

This disease, very common in the southern U. S. in the early 1900s, is still common in parts of the world where corn is the major cereal grain eaten. Corn is deficient in both niacin and tryptophan.

Niacin Use and Misuse

Twenty-five to 50 mg of the vitamin is sufficient to treat a deficiency of niacin.

Large doses of niacin have been suggested to treat schizophrenia and learning disorders in children. In the 1970s, a task force of the American Psychiatric Society reviewed the evidence supporting the use of niacin in the treatment of mental disorders and found that none of the claims could be supported. In spite of this, megavitamin niacin therapy is still recommended for mental illness by some practitioners. There are no scientific studies to support this use or the use of niacin for learning disorders in children.

Large doses of nicotinic acid, in amounts from 500 mg to 3 or 4 grams daily, have been found to lower the level of cholesterol and triglycerides in the blood. Because high levels of blood cholesterol and triglycerides are associated with increased risk of heart attack and stroke, the use of nicotinic acid to treat this condition is becoming increasingly popular. However, side effects may occur when large doses are taken. Doses of 75 mg or more cause blood vessel dilation, which can result in tingling and flushing of the face, neck, and chest. The accompanying itchy skin rash can become painful.

Continued on page 128

Niacin

Niacin Content in Two Daily Diets*

Typical Day's Diet for Woman (1,700 Calories)		Milligrams of Niacin
Breakfast	4 ounces orange juice	0.4
	1 ounce enriched corn flakes	5.0
	1 slice enriched white toast	0.8
	1 pat butter	none
	1 cup 2-percent milk	0.2
	Black coffee	none
Lunch	Sandwich: 2 slices whole-wheat bread, 1 slice American cheese, 2 ounces boiled ham	2.2
	1 cup skim milk (fortified)	0.2
	½ cup cole slaw	0.1
Dinner	½ chicken breast, fried	11.6
	1 medium baked potato	1.3
	1 cup tossed green salad	0.2
	½ cup peas, cooked	1.3
	1 enriched dinner roll	0.9
	2 pats butter	none
	½ cup ice cream	0.5
	Black coffee	none
Total		**24.7**
RDA		**13.0**

*Values for pre-formed niacin. Totals would be higher if tryptophan contribution were included.

Compiled from U.S.D.A. *Home and Garden Bulletin No. 72,* Washington, D.C., revised April 1977.

Niacin Content in Two Daily Diets*

Typical Day's Diet for Teenage Boy (3,000 Calories)		Milligrams of Niacin
Breakfast	½ medium pink grapefruit	0.2
	2 scrambled eggs	none
	2 slices enriched white toast	1.6
	1 pat butter	none
	1 cup whole milk	0.2
Lunch	1 cheeseburger	6.4
	2 cups whole milk	0.4
	10 large French-fried potatoes	1.3
	1 medium banana	0.8
Dinner	4 ounces round steak	6.4
	1 cup green beans	0.2
	1 cup mashed potatoes	2.1
	Lettuce and tomato salad	0.2
	2 slices enriched white bread	1.6
	1 pat butter	none
	1 cup whole milk	0.2
	4 chocolate chip cookies	0.9
Snacks	Cola drink	none
	½ cup ice cream	0.5
	¼ of 14-inch cheese pizza	3.0
Total		**26.0**
RDA		**20.0**

*Values for pre-formed niacin. Totals would be higher if tryptophan contribution were included.

Compiled from U.S.D.A. *Home and Garden Bulletin, No. 72,* Washington, D.C., revised April 1977.

Niacin

Continued from page 125

In addition to the reaction noted earlier, large doses of nicotinic acid can cause indigestion, peptic ulcers, injury to the liver, and an increased blood level of both uric acid and glucose. High blood levels of glucose can be misinterpreted as diabetes, while high levels of uric acid can lead to a misdiagnosis of gout.

High doses of the other form of niacin, niacinamide, have not caused any adverse reactions. However, niacinamide does not lower blood cholesterol and triglycerides.

Daily doses of 150 mg have been prescribed by some headache specialists for the treatment of migraine. The hope is that the dilating effects of niacin will eventually help stabilize the over-dilating/constricting cycle of the patients' cerebral blood vessels. Because of potential side effects, patients are carefully monitored. Without a successful track record to fall back on, and with current reports being inconclusive, most physicians still rely on more conventional methods of treatment.

Pantothenic Acid

Pantothenic acid is everywhere. It occurs in all living cells, and can be found—at least to some extent—in all foods. Although the vitamin was discovered over 40 years ago, it has sparked little interest in nutritionists because a human deficiency of this kind is very rare. In fact, symptoms of vitamin deficiency occur in people only after long periods of food restriction. Nevertheless, some authors of popular books on nutrition blame pantothenic acid deficiency for arthritis, Addison's disease, and allergies. Conversely, others believe the vitamin can improve mental processes, get rid of gray hair, and ensure normal births.

History

Investigators weren't looking for the cause of and cure for a specific human disease when they discovered pantothenic acid in the 1930s. Rather, they were looking for a sustance that was necessary for the growth of yeast. In the process, researchers

Pantothenic Acid

noted that diets lacking the substance they isolated caused certain disorders in animals, and that the symptoms of deficiency varied from species to species. Generally, however, animals who were fed diets without the substance had a retarded growth rate, anemia, degenerated nerve tissue, decreased production of antibodies, ulcers, and malformed off-spring. The newly discovered substance was called pantothenic acid, derived from the Greek word *pantos*, meaning "everywhere."

Since many animal species proved to have a dietary requirement for pantothenic acid, scientists believed that people probably needed it, too. In the 1950s, investigators designed experiments to determine how a diet without pantothenic acid would affect human beings. In the experiments, volunteers were fed a highly purified diet that lacked pantothenic acid, yet contained all the other essential nutrients. After three or four weeks on this diet, the volunteers complained of weakness and an overall "un-well" feeling. One subject had burning cramps.

To accelerate and intensify the deficiency, a few volunteers received the pantothenic acid-deficiency diet plus a compound that specifically interfered with this substance. These subjects developed symptoms faster than those in the other group, and complained of insomnia, depression, gastrointestinal problems, leg cramps, and a burning sensation on the hands and feet. Like those in the original group, these subjects had signs of reduced production of antibodies. In both groups of subjects, all symptoms disappeared after pantothenic acid was administered. Scientists concluded, therefore, that pantothenic acid was an essential vitamin in the human diet.

Function of Pantothenic Acid

Pantothenic acid, formerly called vitamin B_3, is a part of important biologic compounds. One of these, called coenzyme A (CoA), is involved in the release of energy from carbohydrates, fats, and proteins, and in the synthesis of certain compounds. The other— acyl carrier protein (ACP)—participates in the synthesis of fats.

Sources of Pantothenic Acid

All foods contain this vitamin in varying amounts. The best sources are eggs, salmon, liver, kidney, peanuts, wheat bran, and yeast. Fresh vegetables are good sources, and are better than canned vegetables because the canning process decreases the amount of pantothenic acid available. See the table at the end of this profile for food sources of the vitamin.

Dietary Requirements for Pantothenic Acid

The *estimated safe and adequate daily intake* for adults is 4 to 7 mg. It's estimated that the average American gets about 10 to 20 mg in a typical diet.

Continued on page 133

Pantothenic Acid
Content of Common Foods

Food	Quantity	Milligrams of Pantothenic Acid
Meat–Protein Group		
Beef liver, raw	3 ounces	6.55
Beef kidney, raw	3 ounces	3.27
Egg; fresh, raw	1 whole	0.80
Round steak	3 ounces	0.54
Ham, cured	3 ounces	0.48
Almonds; dried, shelled	3½ ounces	0.47
Salmon, canned	3 ounces	0.47
Ground beef	3 ounces	0.37
Pork chop; meat only, cooked	3 ounces	0.34
Liverwurst	1 ounce	0.22
Milk–Dairy Group		
Milk, whole or skim	1 cup	0.84
Cottage cheese	1 cup	0.54
Ice cream	1 cup	0.53
Blue cheese	1 ounce	0.51
Cheddar cheese	1 ounce	0.14
Swiss cheese	1 ounce	0.10
Bread–Cereal/Grain Group		
100% Bran cereal	1 ounce	0.82
40% Bran Flakes cereal	1 ounce	0.25
Bread, whole-wheat	1 slice	0.19
Bread, rye	1 slice	0.13
Bread, white enriched	1 slice	0.11

Pantothenic Acid
Content of Common Foods (continued)

Food	Quantity	Milligrams of Pantothenic Acid
Fruits—Vegetables Group		
Cauliflower, raw	3½ ounces	1.00
Grapefruit	½ medium	0.67
Corn, canned	1 cup	0.56
Banana	1 medium	0.45
Orange	1 medium	0.45
Asparagus, canned	1 cup	0.37
Tomato juice	4 ounces	0.28
Green beans, raw	3½ ounces	0.19
Apple, unpared	1 medium	0.15
Cabbage; shredded, raw	1 cup	0.14
Carrot, raw	1 medium	0.14

Compiled from Orr, M.L., *Pantothenic Acid, Vitamin B$_6$ and Vitamin B$_{12}$ in Foods*, Agricultural Research Service, U.S.D.A., Home Economics Research Report No. 36, Washington, D.C., 1969; and *Lessons on Meat*, National Live Stock and Meat Board, Chicago, 1976.

Continued from page 131

It has also been found that some pantothenic acid is made by bacteria living in the intestine, but it has yet to be determined if this contributes to the body's supply.

Pantothenic Acid

Deficiency of Pantothenic Acid

Pantothenic acid deficiency is not likely to occur when people eat ordinary diets that consist of a variety of foods. Symptoms of deficiency, such as insomnia, leg cramps, or burning feet, have only been seen in experimental situations. Even then, severe symptoms occur only after subjects have been given a drug that interferes with the vitamin.

Pantothenic Acid Use and Misuse

Pantothenic acid isn't used to treat any health problem or condition other than its own deficiency in the rare case of its occurrence.

A deficiency of pantothenic acid in black laboratory rats results in gray hair. This finding lead some people to assume that supplements of the vitamin could prevent people's hair from turning gray. Unfortunately, pantothenic acid does not prevent gray hair from occurring in humans, nor does it reverse the graying process once it has begun.

Cases of toxicity from large doses of pantothenic acid haven't been reported. However, massive doses (10 to 20 g a day) have occasionally caused diarrhea.

Vitamin B$_6$: Pyridoxine

Currently, nutritionists don't know whether Americans get enough vitamin B$_6$ or not. Although there's no evidence of widespread deficiency, some nutritionists believe that the usual intake of the vitamin is just barely enough. However, until large-scale surveys of nutritional status assess vitamin B$_6$ directly, nutritionists can't say for certain whether or not people are actually getting their fair share of this B-complex vitamin.

History

The decade between 1930 and 1940 produced the discovery of one B vitamin after another. In 1933, it was riboflavin; a year later, thiamin. In 1937, it was niacin; then, in 1939, vitamin B$_6$.

Vitamin B$_6$ is not one substance but three: pyridoxine, pyridoxamine, and pyridoxal. All three have the same biologic activity, and all three occur

Continued on page 137

Vitamin B$_6$: Pyridoxine

Sources of Vitamin B$_6$ (Pyridoxine)

Food	Amount	Milli-grams	Percent of U.S. RDA
Most, Kellogg's	1 cup	2.0	100
Tuna, canned	3½ ounces	.90	45
Liver	3 ounces	.84	42
Chicken	3½ ounces	.70	35
Corn Flakes, Kellogg's	1 cup	.70	35
Banana	1 medium	.61	31
Kix, General Mills	1½ cups	.50	25
Avocado	½ medium	.46	23
Pork	3 ounces	.45	23
Beef	3 ounces	.44	22
Halibut	3 ounces	.43	22
Brussel sprouts, cooked	4 large	.40	20
Carnation Instant Breakfast	1 envelope	.40	20
Egg yolk	1	.30	15
Corn, canned	½ cup	.30	15
Sunflower seeds	2 tablespoons	.22	11
Brewer's yeast	1 tablespoon	.20	10
Cottage cheese, creamed	½ cup	.20	10
Asparagus, cooked	½ cup	.20	10
Summer squash, cooked	½ cup	.20	10
Wheat germ	2 tablespoons	.15	8
Frankfurter	1	.14	7
Lima beans, cooked	½ cup	.12	6
Cantaloupe	¼ melon	.12	6
Peanut butter	2 tablespoons	.11	6

Sources of Vitamin B$_6$ (Pyridoxine) (continued)

Food	Amount	Milli-grams	Percent of U.S. RDA
Tomato	1 medium	.10	5
Yogurt	8 ounces	.10	5
Spoon Size Shredded Wheat	1 cup	.10	5
Peanuts	2 tablespoons	.10	5

The RDA for vitamin B$_6$ is 2.2 mg for males, 2.0 mg for females.
The U.S. RDA (labeling tool) for vitamin B$_6$ is 2.0 mg.

Continued from page 135

naturally in food. Plant foods are generally are high in pyridoxine; pyridoxamine and pyridoxal are more common in animal foods. In one form or another, vitamin B$_6$ is found in all food substances.

Function of Pyridoxine

Pyridoxine functions mainly in the metabolism of protein and its component amino acids. It's not directly involved in the release of energy like some other B vitamins. Pyridoxine helps remove the nitrogen from amino acids making them available as sources of energy.

Pyridoxine also helps in the manufacture of other important compounds such as antibodies, hemoglobin, and hormones.

Continued on page 139

Vitamin B₆: Pyridoxine

Vitamin B₆ Content of Common Foods

Food	Quantity	Milligrams of Vitamin B₆
Meat–Protein Group		
Beef liver, raw	3 ounces	0.71
Chicken, uncooked	3 ounces	0.42
Pork chop; meat only, cooked	3 ounces	0.41
Ground beef, cooked	3 ounces	0.39
Round steak, cooked	3 ounces	0.39
Tuna, canned	3 ounces	0.36
Ham	3 ounces	0.30
Salmon, canned	3 ounces	0.25
Egg, fresh	1 whole	0.06
Bread–Cereal/Grain Group		
Ready-to-eat breakfast cereals (enriched)		
Special K, Total	1 ounce each	2.00
Corn flakes, Grape Nuts Flakes, raisin bran, Wheaties	1 ounce each	0.50
Bread, whole-wheat	1 slice	0.04
Bread, white enriched	1 slice	0.01
Milk–Dairy Group		
Cottage cheese	1 cup	0.10
Milk, whole or skim	1 cup	0.10
Cheddar cheese	1 ounce	0.02
Fruits–Vegetables Group		
Banana	1 medium	0.89
Corn, canned	1 cup	0.51
Potato, uncooked	1 medium	0.25

Vitamin B$_6$
Content of Common Foods (continued)

Food	Quantity	Milligrams of Vitamin B$_6$
Fruits–Vegetables Group		
Tomato juice	4 ounces	0.23
Green or snap beans, canned	1 cup	0.17
Lima beans, canned	1 cup	0.15
Spinach, canned	1 cup	0.13
Cabbage; chopped, raw	1 cup	0.11
Orange	1 medium	0.11
Grapefruit	½ medium	0.08
Carrot, raw	1 medium	0.07
Apple, unpared	1 medium	0.05
Potato chips	10 pieces	0.04

Compiled from Orr, M.L., *Pantothenic Acid, Vitamin B$_6$ and Vitamin B$_{12}$ in Foods,* Agricultural Research Service, U.S.D.A., Home Economics Research Report No. 36, Washington, D.C., 1969; and *Lessons on Meat,* National Live Stock and Meat Board, Chicago, 1976.

Continued from page 137

Sources of Pyridoxine

As we said, vitamin B$_6$ occurs in three different forms: pyridoxine, pyridoxamine, and pyridoxal. All three forms appear to have the same biologic activity, and one form or another occurs in all foods.

Wheat, salmon, nuts, wheat germ, brown rice, peas, and beans are good sources. Vegetables contain smaller amounts, but if eaten in large quantities, they can still be an important source. Pyridoxine is not

Vitamin B$_6$: Pyridoxine

regularly added to enriched products, but it is added to some highly fortified cereals.

Dietary Requirements for Pyridoxine

The Recommended Dietary Allowance (RDA) for the vitamin is 2.2 mg for men and 2.0 mg for women. The dietary requirement for pyridoxine is related to the amount of protein eaten since this vitamin functions in protein metabolism. Additional amounts are recommended during pregnancy or nursing. The recommended levels are believed to be sufficient to accommodate the high-protein diet that is common for most Americans.

Deficiency of Pyridoxine

The Nationwide Food Consumption Survey done in 1980 showed that the intake of pyridoxine was below 70 percent of the RDA in half of the people surveyed. This survey didn't evaluate blood levels, but other studies have shown reduced blood levels of pyridoxine in some pregnant women, elderly adults, alcohol abusers, and people with certain disorders like kidney disease and Down's Syndrome. The use of some prescription medications, including birth control pills, steroids, or the antibiotics isoniazid or penicillamine, increases the need for pyridoxine. If a pyridoxine supplement is to be used while taking one of these drugs, the situation should be discussed with your doctor.

Vitamin B$_6$: Pyridoxine

Pyridoxine Use and Misuse

Supplement doses of 10 to 50 mg a day of pyridoxine have been used in people who have a condition such as those listed above which increase the body's need. In addition, some people are born with metabolic errors that increase their need for the vitamin. Supplements of pyridoxine are used in persons with sickle cell anemia.

Pyridoxine supplements have been recommended for many disorders including the nausea of pregnancy, premenstrual symptoms, Chinese Restaurant Syndrome (sensitivity to the flavor enhancer monosodium glutamate), and Carpal Tunnel Syndrome, a condition in which there's painful pressure on nerves in the wrist. Its value in these situations is controversial because of both the lack of supporting data and the potential danger associated with large doses.

There have been reports of toxicity in women taking doses of 500 mg and more of pyridoxine for an extended period of time to reduce symptoms of premenstrual syndrome. (Five hundred milligrams is 250 times the RDA.) These women developed tingling and numbness in their hands and feet and were unable to walk. When they discontinued the supplement, symptoms began to disappear.

Excess pyridoxine has been reported to increase excretion of a substance called oxylate in the urine. This increases the risk of developing kidney stones.

Biotin

"Caution! Egg whites may be hazardous to your health." No, the Surgeon General *has not gone so far as to print that phrase* on egg cartons, and, except for a man who was reported to live on six dozen raw eggs a week, no one is in any real danger. But, almost 50 years ago, raw egg whites caused a real problem for some experimental animals. And the cure for the animals' problem turned out to be an essential nutrient for people.

History

In the 1930s, an investigator at the Lister Institute of Preventive Medicine in London, England, was experimenting with the diets of rats. After feeding the rodents raw egg whites for several weeks, he noticed that the animals developed an eczema-like skin condition, lost their hair, became paralyzed, and began to hemorrhage under their skin.

Later, another team of investigators fed rats different foods to see which ones prevented or alleviated the "egg-white syndrome." Various kinds of foods (such as dried yeast, milk, and egg yolk) were found to cure the rats' condition. When this was discovered, researchers then zeroed in on these foods to find out just what they all had in common.

In 1940, Paul Gyorgy identified the common denominator as a vitamin. At first, thinking that it was an isolated substance, he named it vitamin H. Soon after, scientists found that it was actually a member of the B-complex family, and it was renamed *biotin*.

Function of Biotin

Biotin acts as a coenzyme in several metabolic reactions. It plays a role in the manufacture of body fats, in the metabolism of carbohydrates, and in the conversion of amino acids from protein into sugar.

Sources of Biotin

Milk, liver, egg yolk, yeast, and dried peas and beans are good sources of biotin. Nuts and mushrooms contain smaller amounts of the vitamin. See page 144 for the biotin content in common foods.

Biotin is also made by bacteria in the intestine, thus adding to the body's supply.

Dietary Requirements for Biotin

The *safe and adequate intake* of biotin suggested in Table 2 of the RDA is 100 to 200 μg (micrograms)

Continued on page 144

Biotin

Biotin Content of Common Foods

Food	Quantity	Micrograms of Biotin
Meat—Protein Group		
Beef liver, raw	3½ oz.	100
Frankfurter	1	1
Oysters, raw	3½ oz.	10
Clams, raw	3½ oz.	2
Sardines, in oil	3½ oz.	5
Bread—Cereal/Grain Group		
Bran flakes	¾ cup	3
Raisin Bran	¾ cup	3
Wheat Chex	⅔ cup	2
Milk—Dairy Group		
Skim milk	1 cup	5
Whole milk	1 cup	8
Yogurt	1 cup	3
Blue Cheese	3½ oz	7
Brie	3½ oz	7
Cheddar	3½ oz	3
Cottage Cheese	3½ oz	2
Fruits—Vegetables Group		
Banana	1 medium	4
Grapefruit	½	3
Cauliflower	1 cup	17

Continued from page 143

a day. It's estimated that the typical varied diets eaten by people in the United States provide about 100 to 300 μg. This amount, in addition to that which is produced by intestinal bacteria, should provide a quantity sufficient to meet the needs of healthy people.

Deficiency of Biotin

A deficiency of biotin occurs only in unusual circumstances. For example, people on bizarre diets which include large amounts of raw egg whites have been reported to exhibit symptoms of a deficiency. In these cases, the deficiency results from the fact that raw egg whites contain a substance called *avidin* that combines with biotin and prevents its absorption in the body. Cooking egg whites deactivates this substance.

When antibiotic medications are taken that destroy intestinal bacteria, and a diet regimen is provided that lacks biotin, the possiblity of a biotin deficiency exists.

Some people are born with an inherited disorder that increases their need for biotin. In this situation, a supplement may be needed to prevent a biotin deficiency.

Biotin Use and Misuse

Biotin supplements may be needed in the rare instances cited above.

Large doses of biotin have not been found to be toxic.

Folacin

Research leading to the discovery of folacin was closely related to the investigations that resulted in the discovery of vitamin B_{12}. It was found that these two vitamins work together in several important biologial reactions. A deficiency of either vitamin results in a condition known as megaloblastic or macrocytic (large cell) anemia.

History

As early as 1930, researcher Lucy Wills and her colleagues reported that yeast contained a substance which could cure the macrocytic anemia prevalent among the pregnant women in India, with whom they were working. It wasn't until the early 1940s, however, that the substance—folacin—was isolated and identified.

It was discovered that, in foods, most of the vitamin occurs in several different forms which together are called folacin. Folacin, folic acid, and folate all refer to the same B vitamin. Folic acid is the simplest form of the vitamin. It's found in only small amounts in foods, but it's the form included in most vitamin supplements. The expression "folate activity" is often used to describe the actual biological potency or vitamin value of a food.

Function of Folacin

Folacin functions as a coenzyme in many reactions in the body. It has an important role in making new cells, since it functions in the synthesis of the genetic material DNA (deoxyribonucleic acid) and RNA (ribonucleic acid). These substances carry and transfer (respectively) the genetic material that acts as a blueprint in cell production. Folacin is especially needed in any body tissue (such as the intestine) where new cells are constantly and rapidly being manufactured.

This function of folacin helps to explain why the vitamin is necessary for normal growth and development, and why anemia occurs when there's not enough. Large numbers of red blood cells have to be synthesized each day to replace the red cells that are normally destroyed. Synthesis of DNA is essential for this process.

Sources of Folacin

Folacin is found in green, leafy vegetables like broccoli, spinach, and asparagus. (The name *folacin* is actually derived from the word foliage.) Seeds, liver, and dried peas and beans are other good sources.

Continued on page 149

Folacin

Sources of Folic Acid

Food	Amount	Micro-grams	Percent of U.S. RDA
Product 19, Kellogg's	1 cup	400	100
Brewer's yeast	1 tablespoon	310	76
Orange juice	1 cup	160	40
Romaine lettuce, chopped	1 cup	100	25
Brussels sprouts	3 large	100	25
Carnation Breakfast Bar	1	100	25
Crispix, Kellogg's	¾ cup	100	25
Cocoa Krispies, Kellogg's	1 cup	100	25
Beets	2 medium	90	23
Sweet potato	1 medium	80	20
Asparagus	5-6 spears	60	15
Orange	1 medium	60	15
Wheat germ	¼ cup	50	13
Cantaloupe, diced	1 cup	50	13
Grapefruit juice	½ cup	50	13
Milk, regular	1 cup	40	10
Red pepper	1 medium	40	10
Avocado	½ medium	40	10
Yogurt	8 ounces	30	8
Beer	12 ounces	30	8
Cucumber	1 small	30	8
Cabbage	½ cup	20	5
Potato	1 medium	20	5
Strawberries	1 cup	20	5
Whole-wheat bread	1 slice	20	5

The RDA for folic acid is 400 µg.

The U.S. RDA (labeling tool) for folic acid is 400 µg.

Continued from page 147
Orange juice contains less of the vitamin, but is considered a good source because it also contains vitamin C—and vitamin C actually helps preserve folacin values. Since cooking destroys folacin, orange juice is also considered a good source because it's used in its natural state.

Dietary Requirements for Folacin

The Recommended Dietary Allowance (RDA) for folacin is 400 μg (micrograms) for adults. During pregnancy, 800 μg are recommended, since so many new cells are being made. It has been estimated that the average American diet provides about 200 to 250 μg of the vitamin.

Folacin is found in foods both in free form and bound to amino acids. Folacin must be freed before it can be absorbed. Vitamin B_{12} helps the body use folacin.

Deficiency of Folacin

Folacin deficiency can result from inadequate intake or reduced absorption. It may also occur during periods of increased need such as during multiple pregnancies, cancer, or severe burns.

Some medications can interfere with the body's ability to use this vitamin. These medications include aspirin, oral contraceptives, and certain drugs used to treat convulsions, psoriasis, and cancer. In addi-

Folacin

tion, abuse of alcohol can damage the intestine so that less folacin is absorbed. Symptoms of folacin deficiency include diarrhea, weight loss, anemia, and a red, sore, and swollen tongue. The type of anemia —a macrocytic anemia—caused by folacin deficiency is prevalent in underdeveloped countries among the pregnant women of low-income populations. Macrocytic anemia caused by folacin deficiency is not commonly seen in the United States because of supplement use during pregnancy.

About 10 mg of folacin is stored in the liver of healthy people who eat well-balanced diets. This quantity is enough to last about four to five months.

Folacin Use and Misuse

Over-the-counter vitamin supplements generally contain about 400 μg of folacin, which is the RDA for the vitamin. Excess intake of folacin may actually mask a deficiency of vitamin B_{12} and an underlying anemia, known as pernicious anemia. The large doses of folacin cause the blood to appear normal, which, in turn, may delay diagnosis and treatment, resulting in serious, irreversible damage to the nervous system. The longer the delay, the more serious the damage.

When there's a deficiency of folacin, appropriate doses of the vitamin should be prescribed by a doctor.

Under normal circumstances, large amounts of folacin have not been found to be toxic, but they may interfere with the action of drugs taken to control seizures or others taken to treat cancer. As we said earlier, large amounts of folacin may also cover up and delay diagnosis of pernicious anemia permitting nerve damage to continue unchecked.

Vitamin B$_{12}$: Cyanocobalamin/ Cobalamin

Vitamin B$_{12}$ is unique. It differs from other vitamins, even those of the B-complex, in many ways. The vitamin has a chemical structure much more complex than that of any other. It's the only vitamin to contain an inorganic element (the mineral cobalt) as an integral part of its make-up. Only microorganisms or bacteria can synthesize vitamin B$_{12}$. Plants and animals can't make it.

Vitamin B$_{12}$ can't be absorbed from the intestinal tract without the help of a substance which is made in the stomach—the *intrinsic factor*. The intrinsic factor combines with the vitamin B$_{12}$ that's released from food during digestion. It carries the vitamin to the lower part of the small intestine, where there are special receptor cells that the intrinsic factor recognizes and to which it attaches itself. The vitamin B$_{12}$ is released from its carrier and enters these cells to be absorbed into the body. Without the intrinsic

Vitamin B$_{12}$: Cyanocobalamin/Cobalamin

factor, vitamin B$_{12}$ will miss its connection with the receptor cells and will pass out of the body.

Some people have a condition known as pernicious anemia and can't make the intrinsic factor. They can't absorb vitamin B$_{12}$, even if there's plenty of the vitamin in their diets. Eventually, they show symptoms of a vitamin B$_{12}$ deficiency.

History

The pursuit of vitamin B$_{12}$ began in 1926 when two investigators found that patients who ate almost a pound of raw liver a day were effectively relieved of pernicious anemia. But investigators didn't know why. Scientists speculated that liver must contain some substance that prevents or cures the disorder, but they wondered why victims of pernicious anemia needed it in such large quantities.

Scientist William Castle hypothesized that liver contained an antipernicious anemia (APA) factor necessary to treat the anemia. He also believed that people who had the disease lacked an internal or intrinsic factor necessary to use the APA. By eating about a pound of liver a day, these people could counteract the lack of the intrinsic factor and absorb the APA they needed.

For the next 20 years, scientists searched for the APA. Research was time consuming since experimental animals were not suitable for the testing required. Instead, testing had to be performed over long

Vitamin B$_{12}$: Cyanocobalamin/Cobalamin

periods of time on human subjects. For these experiments, scientists prepared extracts of liver and separated them into different fractions. Then, each fraction was given to someone with pernicious anemia, and the researchers had to wait for a change, to see which fraction, if any, contained the APA.

Progress was slow until 1948, when an "experimental animal" was found that could be used for testing—the microorganism, *Lactobacillus lactus Dorner* (LLD). Instead of testing liver extracts on people, researchers tested them on LLD. Since they reproduce so quickly, many generations could be tested in a short period of time.

In less than a year, two research groups—one in England and one in the United States—found the answer. These groups managed to isolate pure vitamin B$_{12}$. As a matter of fact, they extracted about 20 mg of the vitamin from a *ton* of liver. And it turned out that vitamin B$_{12}$ was the APA factor.

Function of Vitamin B$_{12}$

Vitamin B$_{12}$ is essential to cells. It's needed for the synthesis of DNA (deoxyribonucleic acid) and RNA (ribonucleic acid), which transmit and carry (respectively) the data bank of genetic information for every living cell. This information tells a cell how to function and must be passed along each time a cell divides. Rapidly dividing cells need a continuous supply of vitamin B$_{12}$. This vitamin works along with the vitamin folacin in this important role.

Vitamin B_{12}: Cyanocobalamin/Cobalamin

Vitamin B_{12} helps maintain normal bone marrow. It also functions in the production of a material called *myelin*, which covers and protects nerve fibers.

Sources of Vitamin B_{12}

Vitamin B_{12} is found largely in animal foods like liver, meat, clams, oysters, sardines, and salmon. Fermented bean products like tempeh contain some B_{12}. Vitamin B_{12} is also added to some cereals. Bacteria in the intestine make some of the vitamin, but far less than the amount needed daily is absorbed. See the table on pages 156-157 for a list of food sources of vitamin B_{12}.

Dietary Requirements for Vitamin B_{12}

The Recommended Dietary Allowance (RDA) for vitamin B_{12} is 3 μg (micrograms) daily for adults and 4 μg daily for women who are pregnant or breast-feeding. It's estimated that the average diet eaten by Americans provides 7 to 30 μg of the vitamin—more than enough to meet the daily need.

Deficiency of Vitamin B_{12}

When the supply of vitamin B_{12} in the body is low, it slows down the production of red blood cells (causing anemia) and cells that line the intestine. These events are similar to those that occur as a result of

Continued on page 157

Vitamin B$_{12}$: Cyanocobalamin/Cobalamin

Sources of Vitamin B$_{12}$

Food	Amount	Micro-grams	Percent of U.S. RDA
Liver, beef	3½ ounces	80.0	1,300
Liver, chicken	3½ ounces	24.1	400
Clams, canned	½ cup	20.0	333
Oysters, raw	3½ ounces	18.0	300
Liverwurst	2 slices	9.2	153
Crabmeat, canned	3½ ounces	8.5	142
Sardines	3½ ounces	8.3	138
Salmon, canned	3½ ounces	7.5	125
Product 19, Kellogg's	1 cup	6.0	100
Tuna fish	3½ ounces	3.0	50
Morningstar Farms sausages	3	2.4	40
Beefsteak	3 ounces	2.2	36
Hamburger	3 ounces	1.8	30
Veal, lean	3½ ounces	1.8	30
Haddock	3½ ounces	1.7	28
Lamb	3½ ounces	1.6	27
Kix, General Mills	1½ cups	1.5	25
Yogurt	8 ounces	1.3	22
Flounder	3½ ounces	1.2	20
Milk	1 cup	1.0	17
Ham	3½ ounces	.8	13
Cottage cheese	½ cup	.7	12
Egg	1	.6	10
Carnation Breakfast Bar	1	.6	10
Buttermilk	8 ounces	.5	8
Swiss cheese*	1 ounce	.5	8

Vitamin B$_{12}$: Cyanocobalamin/Cobalamin

Sources of Vitamin B$_{12}$ (continued)

Food	Amount	Micro-grams	Percent of U.S. RDA
Bleu cheese*	1 ounce	.4	6
Camembert cheese*	1 ounce	.4	6
Cheddar cheese*	1 ounce	.3	5

The RDA for vitamin B$_{12}$ is 3 µg.

The U.S. RDA (labeling tool) for vitamin B$_{12}$ is 6 µg.

*As cheese ripens, the amount of B vitamins increases.

Continued from page 155

folacin deficiency. But, unlike folacin deficiency, a lack of vitamin B$_{12}$ can also cause serious damage to the nervous system. If the condition persists for a long time, the damage is not reversible.

Deficiencies of vitamin B$_{12}$ caused by eating a diet low in the vitamin are not common. The average well-fed person has a supply of the vitamin stored in the liver that can last five years or longer.

A dietary deficiency of vitamin B$_{12}$ is seen only in strict vegetarians who don't eat foods of animal origin—not even milk or eggs. This very restricted diet poses a particular problem in pregnant or breast-feeding women since the baby can develop a deficiency even when the mother is healthy. All vegetarian mothers should use vitamin B$_{12}$-fortified foods. Vegetarians who eat eggs and/or drink milk get all the vitamin B$_{12}$ they need in their diet.

Vitamin B$_{12}$: Cyanocobalamin/Cobalamin

Pernicious anemia is usually an inherited disease in which a deficiency of vitamin B$_{12}$ occurs, but it's not caused by a lack of the vitamin in the diet. Some people cannot make the intrinsic factor, a substance needed for the absorption of vitamin B$_{12}$, so that even when their diets contain adequate amounts of the vitamin, it's just not absorbed. When this condition exists, vitamin B$_{12}$ must be provided by injection so that it bypasses the stomach and does not depend on the intrinsic factor for absorption.

Partial or total removal of the stomach will also reduce absorption of vitamin B$_{12}$ because the production of intrinsic factor occurs in the stomach. Removal of the ileum portion of the small intestine can also result in deficiency of the vitamin because that's the area where absorption of this vitamin takes place. In these situations, pernicious anemia is the result of surgery.

Vitamin B$_{12}$ Use and Misuse

Pernicious anemia is treated with an injection of 50 to 100 μg of vitamin B$_{12}$ three times a week until symptoms subside. Injections of the vitamin may be needed throughout life to maintain improvement.

Injections of vitamin B$_{12}$ are often used as a tonic or placebo. The vitamin in its crystal form has a bright red color, which apparently adds to the impression that it will help improve well being. Its use for this purpose is controversial.

Vitamin B$_{12}$: Cyanocobalamin/Cobalamin

There are no reports of vitamin B$_{12}$ causing any toxicity or adverse effects even when taken in large amounts. Taking the vitamin orally, however, will not help those people with undiagnosed pernicious anemia as they will not be able to absorb it.

Vitamin C: Ascorbic Acid

When asked what's the first thing that comes into their heads when they hear "vitamin C," many people respond "Linus Pauling" or "the common cold." Although they might not agree with him, most people have heard of Pauling and his book, *Vitamin C and the Common Cold.*

In his 1970 book, Pauling recommended megadoses of vitamin C to reduce the frequency and severity of colds. The book triggered a sales boom for vitamin C. It also prompted nutritionists to begin a series of carefully designed studies of the vitamin. Today, some people still swear by vitamin C even though nutritionists have found little proof of its effectiveness against the common cold.

History

If you recall from the introduction of this book, the story of vitamin C began centuries before the discovery of the vitamin, with accounts of a disease called scurvy.

Scurvy—an ailment characterized by muscle weakness, lethargy, and bleeding under the skin—has been rampant around the world throughout the centuries. Documents dating back before the time of Christ describe the disease. Ships' logs tell of its widespread occurrence among sailors in the 16th century. History books report that scurvy was a common problem among the troops during the American Civil War. And records of Antarctic explorers recount how Captain Robert Scott and his team succumbed to the malady in 1912.

Almost as old as the reports of the disease are the reports of successful ways of treating it. Over the centuries, references were made to the curative properties of green salads, fruits, vegetables, pickled cabbage, small onions, and an ale made of such things as wormwood, horseradish, and mustard seed. In the 1530s, the French explorer, Jacques Cartier, told how Newfoundland Indians cured the disease by giving his men an extract prepared from the green shoots of an evergreen tree.

The disease was still the "scourge of the navy" 200 years later when the British physician James Lind began an experiment that singled out, once and for all, a cure for scurvy. Believing that acidic materials would relieve symptoms of the illness, Lind tried six different substances on six groups of scurvy-stricken men. He gave them all the standard shipboard diet, but to one pair of men in each of the six groups he

Vitamin C: Ascorbic Acid

gave a different test substance. One pair received a solution of sulfuric acid each day; another, cider; and a third, sea water. The fourth pair received vinegar, and the fifth took a daily combination of garlic, mustard seed, balsam of Peru, and gum myrrh. The sixth pair received two oranges and a lemon each day.

Lind found that the men who ate citrus fruit improved rapidly; one was able to return to duty after only six days. The sailors who drank the cider showed slight improvement after two weeks, but those who had received the other test substances did not improve. Although Lind soon published the results of his experiment, 50 years passed before the British navy finally added lime juice to its sailors' diets.

Following the discovery of the cure for scurvy, the next chapter in the story of vitamin C ended in 1932 with the isolation of the vitamin itself by C.G. King and W.A. Waugh at the University of Pittsburgh, and by Albert Szent-Gyorgyi in Hungary.

At the time Szent-Gyorgyi isolated the vitamin, he knew little of its chemical makeup. He only knew that it exhibited some similarities to sugar. He first proposed that the vitamin be given the name ignose, from the Latin *ignosco* for "I do not know," and *ose*, the suffix applied to sugars. The editor of a British scientific journal would not accept the name, so Szent-Gyorgyi suggested an alternative: godnose. When Szent-Gyorgyi's article was finally published in the journal, the vitamin carried the name hexuronic acid. Later the name was changed to ascorbic (meaning "without scurvy") acid.

Vitamin C: Ascorbic Acid

Function of Vitamin C

A major function of vitamin C involves its role as a cofactor in the formation and repair of collagen, a connective tissue that holds the body's cells and tissues together. Vitamin C also promotes the normal development of bones and teeth. It's needed for amino acid metabolism and the synthesis of hormones, including the thyroid hormone that controls the rate of metabolism in the body.

Vitamin C aids the absorption of iron and calcium. Vitamin C is also an antioxidant. This means it protects other substances from being damaged by oxidation (the combining of a substance with oxygen) by combining with oxygen itself. This function makes it a useful food additive in frozen fruits, cured meats and other processed foods. In cured meats, vitamin C inhibits the formation of nitrosamines, compounds that have been shown to cause cancer in laboratory animals.

Sources of Vitamin C

Citrus fruits, such as oranges, lemons, grapefruit, and limes, are excellent sources. Other good sources of vitamin C are strawberries, cantaloupe, and peppers. Potatoes also supply some vitamin C, and this contribution is considered important because of the large amounts of potatoes that are consumed. Rose hips gathered from rose bushes are rich in vitamin C and are often used to prepare a nutritious tea.

Continued on page 169

Vitamin C: Ascorbic Acid

Sources of Vitamin C

Food	Quantity	Percent of U.S. RDA
Currants; black, European, raw	1 cup	550.00
Strawberries, frozen	1 carton (10 ounces)	250.00
Brussels sprouts, cooked	1 cup	225.00
Orange juice, fresh	1 cup	206.67
Orange juice; frozen concentrate, diluted	1 cup	200.00
Lemon juice, fresh	1 cup	186.67
Orange-grapefruit juice; frozen concentrate, diluted	1 cup	170.00
Papayas, raw	1 cup (½-inch cubes)	170.00
Orange juice; canned, unsweetened	1 cup	166.67
Grapefruit juice; frozen concentrate, unsweetened, diluted	1 cup	160.00
Green peppers; sweet, raw (without stem or seeds)	1 pod (⅕ pound)	156.67
Grapefruit juice, fresh	1 cup	153.33
Cantaloupe	½ medium	150.00
Honeydew melon	½ medium	148.33
Strawberries, raw	1 cup	146.67
Collards, cooked	1 cup	145.00
Grapefruit juice; canned, white, unsweetened	1 cup	140.00
Lime juice, fresh	1 cup	131.67
Grapefruit, canned in syrup	1 cup	126.67

Sources of Vitamin C (continued)

Food	Quantity	Percent of U.S. RDA
Broccoli, cooked	½ cup	116.67
Peppers; sweet, boiled, drained	1 pod	116.67
Cress; garden, raw	3½ ounces	115.00
Kale, cooked (leaves, stems)	1 cup	113.33
Mustard greens, cooked	1 cup	113.33
Turnip greens, cooked	1 cup	113.33
Cauliflower, cooked	1 cup	110.00
Oranges, raw (all varieties)	1 orange (2⅝-inch diameter)	110.00
Dandelion greens, raw	1 cup	105.00
Raspberries; red, frozen	1 carton (10 ounces)	98.33
Tangerine juice; canned, sweetened	1 cup	91.67
Lime juice; canned unsweetened	1 cup	86.67
Casaba melon	½ medium	83.33
Spinach, cooked	1 cup	83.33
Cabbage, cooked (common varieties)	1 cup	80.00
Grapefruit, raw	½ medium	73.33
Avocado, raw (late summer, fall: Florida)	1 whole	71.67
Cabbage; red, raw	1 cup	71.67
Cabbage, raw (common variety)	1 cup	70.00
Kale; boiled, drained	1 cup	70.00

Continued on next page

Vitamin C: Ascorbic Acid

Sources of Vitamin C (continued)

Food	Quantity	Percent of U.S. RDA
Tomatoes, raw	1 tomato (3-inch diameter)	70.00
Tomatoes, canned (solids and liquid)	1 cup	68.33
Cranberry juice cocktail, canned	1 cup	66.67
Orange-apricot juice drink	1 cup	66.67
Potato sticks	3 ½ ounces	66.67
Cabbage; savoy, raw	1 cup	65.00
Lemon, raw	1 (2⅛-inch diameter)	65.00
Tomato juice, canned	1 cup	65.00
Asparagus; green, canned	1 cup	61.67
Elderberries, raw	3½ ounces	60.00
Strawberry pie	1 sector	56.67
Turnips; cooked, diced	1 cup	56.67
Peas; green, cooked	1 cup	55.00
Sauerkraut, canned (solids and liquid)	1 cup	55.00
Dandelion greens, cooked	1 cup	53.33
Raspberries; red, raw	1 cup	51.67
Avocado, raw (mid-late winter: California)	1 whole	50.00
Blackberries, raw	1 cup	50.00
Sweet potatoes, canned	1 cup	50.00
Watermelon, raw	1 wedge (4 by 8 inches)	50.00
Beans; lima, cooked, drained	1 cup	48.33

Sources of Vitamin C (continued)

Food	Quantity	Percent of U.S. RDA
Cole slaw with French dressing (commercial)	3½ ounces	48.33
French dressing (homemade)	3½ ounces	48.33
Lettuce; raw, iceberg	1 head (4¾-inch diameter)	48.33
Mayonnaise	3½ ounces	48.33
Cowpeas, cooked	1 cup	46.67
Peaches; dried, uncooked	1 cup	46.67
Tangerines, raw	1 medium	45.00
Winter squash; baked, mashed	1 cup	45.00
Cabbage; spoon or bok choy, cooked	1 cup	43.33
Sweet potatoes, boiled (peeled after boiling)	1 medium	41.67
Cherries; sweet, raw	1 cup	40.00
Pineapple; raw, diced	1 cup	40.00
Spinach, canned (drained solids)	1 cup	40.00
Sweet potatoes, baked (peeled after baking)	1 medium	40.00
Beef liver, fried	3 ounces	38.33
Cucumbers; raw, pared	1 cucumber (10 ounces)	38.33
Beet greens; cooked, drained (leaves and stems)	1 cup	36.67
Peas; green, canned	1 cup	36.67

Continued on next page

Vitamin C: Ascorbic Acid

Sources of Vitamin C (continued)

Food	Quantity	Percent of U.S. RDA
Pineapple juice, canned	1 cup	36.67
Spaghetti with meat balls, tomato sauce (homemade)	1 cup	36.67
Summer squash; cooked, diced	1 cup	35.00
Blueberries, raw	1 cup	33.33
Potatoes, baked (peeled after baking)	1 medium	33.33
Potatoes, boiled (peeled before boiling)	1 medium	33.33
Apricot halves; dried, uncooked	1 cup	31.67
Cabbage; celery or Chinese, raw	1 cup	31.67
Potatoes, mashed (milk added)	1 cup	31.67
Lettuce; Boston, raw	1 head (4-inch diameter)	30.00
Lettuce, cos or romaine	3½ ounces	30.00
Potatoes, mashed (milk and butter added)	1 cup	30.00
Tomato-vegetable soup with noodles, dehydrated	1 package (2½-ounces)	30.00
Leeks, raw (bulb and lower leaf)	3½ ounces	28.33
Lemonade concentrate, diluted	1 cup	28.33
Okra, cooked	8 pods	28.33

Sources of Vitamin C (continued)

Food	Quantity	Percent of U.S. RDA
Rhubarb, cooked (sugar added)	1 cup	28.33
Soybeans; boiled, drained	3½ ounces	28.33
Sweet potatoes, candied	1 potato	28.33
Asparagus; cooked, drained	4 spears	26.67
Parsnips, cooked	1 cup	26.67
Beans; snap, green; cooked, drained	1 cup	25.00
Beef and vegetable stew	1 cup	25.00
Lobster salad	3 ounces	25.00
Spanish rice (homemade)	3½ ounces	25.00
Tomato soup; canned, condensed (with equal amount milk)	1 cup	25.00

Compiled from CONSUMER GUIDE® magazine Nutrition Data Bank.

Continued from page 163

Fruit juices, fruit juice drinks, and drink mixes are often fortified with vitamin C at fairly high levels. See the table on pages 164-169 for sources of vitamin C.

More than any other vitamin, vitamin C can be easily destroyed. The amount in foods decreases rapidly during transport, processing, storage, and preparation. Bruising or cutting a fruit or vegetable will destroy some of the vitamin, as will light, air, and heat. In spite of this, orange juice that is covered and refrigerated will retain much of its vitamin C value

Vitamin C: Ascorbic Acid

even after several days. Even potato chips retain some of the vitamin C that was in the raw potato. However, for maximum vitamin value, it's usually best to use fresh, unprocessed fruits and vegetables whenever possible.

Dietary Requirements for Vitamin C

The Recommended Dietary Allowance (RDA) for vitamin C is 60 mg daily for adults, with an additional 20 mg for pregnant women and an additional 40 mg for women who are breast-feeding. These amounts are several times the amount needed to treat deficiency symptoms, yet some people believe these levels are not high enough. An intake of 100 mg will generally saturate the tissues of most people, and at that point, any additional vitamin C will be excreted in the urine.

Deficiency of Vitamin C

The classic vitamin C deficiency disease is scurvy; in fact, as we said, the name ascorbic acid means "without scurvy." Early signs of the disease are bleeding gums and bleeding under the skin. The deficiency can progress to a point where there's poor wound healing, anemia, and disturbed bone growth and maintenance.

Only 10 mg of vitamin C is needed daily to prevent scurvy, so the disease is seldom seen today, except

Continued on page 172

Vitamin C Content
of Common Foods*

Food	Quantity	Milligrams of Vitamin C
Fruits		
Cantaloupe	½ melon	90
Orange	1 medium	66
Orange juice; frozen, diluted	4 ounces	60
Grapefruit	½ medium	44
Strawberries, fresh	½ cup	44
Banana	1 medium	12
Apple	1 medium	6
Vegetables		
Broccoli; chopped, cooked	½ cup	70
Cauliflower; chopped, raw	½ cup	45
Potato, baked	1 medium	31
Tomato, raw	1 medium	28
Tomato juice, canned	4 ounces	20
Asparagus, cooked	½ cup	19
Cabbage; shredded, raw	½ cup	17
Potato, mashed	½ cup	10
Green or snap beans, cooked	½ cup	8
Carrot, raw	1 medium	6

* *Milk and milk products, cereal foods (unless fortified), and meats contain little or no ascorbic acid. Organ meats are exceptions. Beef liver contains 23 mg ascorbic acid in a three-ounce serving.*

Compiled from product labels and U.S.D.A. *Home and Garden Bulletin No. 72,* Washington, D.C., revised April 1977.

Vitamin C: Ascorbic Acid

Continued from page 170

in infants who are not given a source of vitamin C. Studies show that some male teens and elderly men have low intakes of the vitamin, yet they do not have the disease.

People who smoke cigarettes and women who use oral contraceptives have been shown to have lower than normal blood levels of vitamin C. The RDA level of vitamin C, however, provides enough to meet even these additional needs.

The body normally stores about 1,500 mg of vitamin C, and symptoms do not occur until the body pool is less than 300 mg. It would take several weeks on a diet containing no vitamin C for this drop to occur.

Vitamin C Use and Misuse

Supplements of vitamin C are used to treat deficiency of the vitamin. Vitamin C is also used to acidify the urine during certain bladder or kidney disorders. Sometimes vitamin C supplements are given to people who will be undergoing surgery to ensure that there's a sufficient supply of the vitamin to promote healing.

Vitamin C is one of the most popular vitamins. It has been recommended for cold prevention and for the treatment of schizophrenia, senility, cancer, and other medical problems. For some disorders, it's hard to separate the true effects of the vitamin from the psychological effects. A person taking vitamin C supplements may feel better simply because he or she believes the vitamin is of some benefit.

Scientifically controlled studies testing the value of vitamin C in relation to cold prevention or treatment have shown only a slight beneficial effect in reducing a cold's severity. It appears that the vitamin may act as an antihistamine. For the most part, however, the studies did not prove that large amounts of the vitamin prevented a cold.

A study testing the value of 10 grams a day of vitamin C in cancer patients showed no effect on symptoms or on length of survival.

Large single doses of vitamin C have not been found to be toxic, but continued large intakes have been reported to cause problems. Some people develop cramps and diarrhea when taking 1000 mg or more a day. An interesting aside to this fact is that some believers feel that the onset of diarrhea is an indication that the person is taking sufficient amounts of vitamin C to be effective!

Large doses of vitamin C has been reported to cause the breakdown of red blood cells in people with an inherited disease that makes their blood cells particularly susceptible to the reducing effects of vitamin C. Those with sickle cell anemia have abnormal hemoglobin protein that can be distorted by vitamin C. If this occurs, the protein's shape is changed, causing it to clog blood vessels. For this reason, people with sickle cell anemia should not take large amounts of vitamin C.

Vitamin C: Ascorbic Acid

Others who have taken supplements greater than 1,000 mg a day develop rebound scurvy when they discontinue use. It seems that their bodies have developed mechanisms for breaking down and excreting the vitamin quickly so that a deficiency develops when they begin taking smaller amounts. Scurvy has also been reported in babies whose mothers took large amounts of vitamin C during pregnancy. Apparently, the babies had an increased requirement for the vitamin due to their exposure to extra amounts before birth.

It's recommended that people who have been taking large amounts of vitamin C wean themselves gradually from it rather than just stopping abruptly. This way the body can become accustomed to lower intakes very gradually over a longer period of time.

It's suspected that some susceptible people might develop calcium oxylate kidney stones after taking large doses of vitamin C. The oxylate compound is formed in the metabolism of the vitamin, and may promote stone formation.

Large doses of vitamin C can also result in increased excretion of uric acid. This can be a problem for people who suffer from gout. It can also lead to a misdiagnosis of this condition.

Chewable vitamin tablets containing high levels of vitamin C may erode tooth enamel if used over a long period of time. Large doses of vitamin C may also interfere with the action of some anticlotting medications.

Vitamin C: Ascorbic Acid

Vitamin C is chemically similar to glucose so that when there's a large intake of the vitamin, laboratory tests for the presence of glucose in the urine may be misinterpreted. This may create problems monitoring blood glucose levels in people with diabetes. Large amounts of vitamin C may also cover up the presence of blood in the stool. This can distort the results of tests designed to detect colon cancer.

Chapter 6
Vitaminlike Substances

There are other compounds that are sometimes grouped with the vitamins (and sometimes even called vitamins) because they function in the body in some of the same ways. They do not, however, really fit the definition for vitamins because they're either synthesized in the body or they're needed in larger amounts than vitamins. They're found so widely in foods that a deficiency is unlikely. Choline, bioflavonoids, inositol, lipoic acid, carnitine, coenzyme Q, and para-aminobenzoic acid are some of these vitaminlike substances. There's a possibility that some day when there's more information about them, their status may be changed.

Choline

Choline is a substance found in most animal tissues, either in a free form or a combined form. In combination, it may exist as part of a substance called lecithin, a yellowish or brownish waxy material found in nervous tissue, especially in the protective myelin sheath that surrounds nerve fibers. Or, it may also exist as acetylcholine, a substance essential for the transmission of nerve impulses.

It was discovered that a lack of choline in experimental animals whose pancreases were removed resulted in a condition known as fatty liver or hepatic cirrhosis. When present, choline prevented the fatty degenerative changes that would otherwise occur. It's been suggested that choline supplements might be used for the prevention of this condition in humans. Other equally controversial issues involve the use of choline to lower cholesterol levels and improve memory.

Large doses of choline and lecithin have been used as drugs with a limited degree of success in the treatment of certain conditions. One of those conditions is Alzheimer's disease. Another is tardive dyskinesia, a syndrome marked by involuntary movements, especially of the face and jaw, that results from long-term use of drugs used to treat mental illness and other disorders.

Egg yolks, liver, beef, and soybeans are good sources of choline. Choline can also be made in the body. Under normal circumstances, choline or lecithin supplements are not necessary.

Bioflavonoids

Bioflavonoids are found in citrus fruits and their skins. In the 1930s, bioflavonoids were believed to be essential to human nutrition because it was thought that they could reverse the effects of vitamin C deficiency. This idea was later proven to be incorrect. At the present time, there is no evidence that bioflavonoids are essential.

Although many claims have been made for the use of bioflavonoids for bleeding problems, strokes, and joint disease, they have not been documented.

Inositol

Inositol is found in liver, wheat germ, citrus fruits, and meat. It can also be synthesized in the body and is found especially in hair and muscles. It has been suggested as a treatment for baldness, but there's no evidence that it's effective for this use. Its function is not yet completely understood, but it's believed to be involved in the metabolism of fats.

Lipoic Acid

Lipoic acid functions as a coenzyme along with the vitamin thiamin. Yeast and liver are good sources of this substance, but it can also be synthesized by the body.

Carnitine (Vitamin B-T)

Carnitine plays a role in fat and energy metabolism in the body. Recently, carnitine has received publicity as being useful for people with heart disease. However, more research is needed to establish its value, if any, for heart patients. Carnitine is found in greater amounts in foods of animal origin and lesser amounts in foods of plant origin, so that a vegetarian diet is apt to be low in carnitine. But, since, under normal circumstances, this substance is synthesized in the body, this is of little concern.

Coenzyme Q

Coenzyme Q, also called ubiquinone, is chemically related to vitamin E. Coenzyme Q is synthesized by the body and plays a role in energy metabolism. Current research is examining the benefit of coenzyme Q supplements in the treatment of certain types of heart disease.

Para-Aminobenzoic Acid (PABA)

PABA is part of the B vitamin folacin and, therefore, isn't considered a separate vitamin. PABA is used in sunscreens and, when applied to the skin, can serve to protect against sunburn. Taken orally, however, PABA does not have the same effect. Large doses taken over extended periods of time can cause nausea and vomiting.

Chapter 7

The Story of Minerals

Ancient people recognized the value and usefulness of minerals. We can see this in the following examples:

- Chinese writings from as early as 3,000 B.C. described the condition known as goiter, and recommended seaweed and burnt sponge to treat it. Goiter is caused by a deficiency of the mineral iodine, and both seaweed and sponges are rich in this mineral.

- In ancient Greece, people soaked hot iron swords in water and then used the iron-enriched water to treat anemia.

- As many as 30 references to salt (a compound composed of two minerals—sodium and chlorine) can be found in the Bible, including its use in purifying ceremonies and as an offering to God.

- A Greek slave, who was said to be "worth his weight in salt," was actually bought for a certain quantity of this substance.

- At banquets, important people were asked to sit in a position at the table that placed them closest to the salt cellar. This was considered a position of honor.

- The word *salary* comes from the Latin word for salt, "saleria."

Despite all of these early references to the use of minerals, many centuries passed before researchers could clarify the role that minerals play in the body. In 1799, the French chemist Antoine Lavoisier (often called the "father of nutrition") correctly predicted that "elements," known today as minerals, would soon be isolated from the "earths."

In 1804, another Frenchman, Theodore de Saussure, proved that the nature of the soil influenced the mineral content of plants grown on that soil.

By the beginning of the 19th century, scientists were beginning to gather knowledge on the nature of minerals. Research on minerals continued in the second half of the 19th century with much work being done on trace minerals—those only needed in tiny amounts. And by the end of the century, a few of the minerals now known to be important were actually understood.

In the early 20th century, as vitamins were being isolated and their importance identified, many minerals were also shown to be essential to human nutrition. It's been calculated that minerals, sometimes referred to as inorganic elements, make up about 4 percent of the body's weight—or the equivalent of about five pounds. About 50 different minerals have been found in the body, and of these, it's estimated that about 17 are actually essential, while the others are there as accidental contaminants. This estimate may be somewhat low since its been recently shown, for example, that boron, one of the so-called accidental contaminants, has been linked to the metabolism of minerals and may even be a factor in bone development. It's possible that some of the other members of this category may prove to be useful to the body as well.

What Are Minerals?

Minerals are different from the vitamins discussed in the first part of the book because minerals are not organic substances made by plants or animals. They're actually inorganic elements found in the soil. Plants absorb minerals directly from the soil, and animals get their supply indirectly, by eating the plants or by eating other animals who have eaten the plants.

Minerals are grouped into two categories depending upon the amount that is normally found in the body. Those that are found in significant amounts are called *macrominerals*. These include calcium, phosphorus, magnesium, chlorine, sodium, potassium, and sulfur. Generally, the body contains about five grams or more of each of these minerals. Calcium and phosphorus occur in the largest amounts—about one pound or more.

The Story of Minerals

The other category of minerals is the *microminerals*. This group consists of the *trace elements* that are found in the body in smaller amounts. In fact, the daily requirement for these minerals is only a few milligrams or less. Among the microminerals that have been determined to be essential to humans are iron, iodine, zinc, fluoride, copper, chromium, manganese, selenium, molybdenum, and cobalt.

Research continues to suggest that there may be other trace minerals such as nickel, tin, silicon, and vanadium that are essential for animals. It's possible that these may prove to be necessary for humans as well. Arsenic, cadmium, boron, aluminum, and lead are referred to as trace contaminants because, although they are found in the body, they are not currently believed to be essential. In the future, some or all of these may be found to serve important roles. At the present time, however, there's actually concern about exposure to contaminants such as lead, cadmium, mercury, and arsenic, since they've been found to be particularly toxic when present in excess amounts.

The National Research Council has established Recommended Dietary Allowances (RDAs) for six minerals: calcium, iron, phosphorus, magnesium, zinc, and iodine. Ranges of safe and adequate daily intakes have been established for sodium, chlorine, copper, fluoride, chromium, selenium, manganese, and molybdenum. Since there's less information available about this latter group, more precise recommendations are not possible. In the table *Estimated Safe and Adequate Daily Dietary Intakes of Additional*

The Story of Minerals

Selected Vitamins and Minerals (see pages 26-27) where these suggested intakes are presented, there's also a footnote warning about the habitual intake of excessive amounts.

What Minerals Do

Minerals function as structural components of living tissue and as regulators of important processes that occur in the body. They're found in every cell and are involved in some way with almost everything the body does.

In their structural role, minerals contribute strength and firmness to bones and teeth. They're also part of essential body compounds. For example, iron is a part of hemoglobin (the oxygen-carrying substance in the blood), iodine is a part of thyroid hormone, and cobalt is a part of vitamin B_{12}. In their role as regulators, minerals act as cofactors in enzyme-controlled metabolic reactions that occur within the body.

Free mineral ions, which are particles that have either a positive or negative electrical charge, have many important functions. They include maintenance of normal water balance and acid-base balance, transmission of nerve impulses, regulation of normal cell membrane function, regulation of muscle response to stimuli, and start-up mechanisms for enzyme systems.

Some minerals have been shown to have drug-like effects. For example, fluoride has been shown to prevent tooth decay, and lithium salts have been used to treat mental illness. Lithium, however, is not one of the minerals we'll be discussing, since it's not normally found in the body.

Mineral Deficiencies

Major nutrition surveys often find that intakes of certain minerals, such as calcium and iron, are lower than the RDAs in many population groups.

Foods that are refined and processed tend to have fewer minerals. To remedy this, minerals may be added to replace those lost in processing, or may be added simply for fortification. As early as the 1920s, iodine was added to salt to prevent or treat iodine deficiency. Iron is added routinely to enrich cereals and breads. Recently, calcium is being added to fruit juices and dry breakfast cereals.

Mineral Toxicity

Taking large doses of mineral supplements can be harmful. Large doses may cause abnormal fluid accumulations in body organs or may interfere with the body's use of other minerals.

A Word About Water

In the body, metabolic reactions involving vitamins and minerals take place in water. Thus, water is es-

The Story of Minerals

sential for the maintenance of normal body function. Water makes up about 60 percent of an adult's body and an even greater percentage of a child's body. About 70 percent of lean body tissue is actually water. Water carries nutrients and wastes, respectively, into and out of cells. It acts as a solvent for compounds such as vitamins, minerals, glucose, and amino acids (the building blocks of protein). It lubricates joints, acts as a shock absorber inside the eye and spinal cord, and aids the body in maintaining its temperature.

The average daily intake of water is about 2½ quarts. Normally, this amount is obtained from many sources. Some of our supply comes from drinks (such as milk, water, coffee, tea, soft drinks, and soups), foods of animal origin (such as meat, fish, or eggs), and fruits and vegetables. For example, it's estimated that cucumbers contain about 96 percent water, lettuce 94 percent, watermelon 93 percent, broccoli 91 percent, and oranges 84 percent. Water is also formed in the body as a by-product of metabolism.

Water is also *lost* from the body each day. It's lost in urine, stool, sweat, and in the air we exhale. (You can see that we exhale water by observing the mist that forms on a mirror or a pair of glasses when you blow on them, or by noticing the water vapor that looks like a puff of steam coming out of your mouth on a day when the temperature is below 32°F [0°C].) People who are healthy generally excrete at least one quart of urine a day to get rid of body wastes. During the waking hours, this can mean that people may urinate approximately every four hours. Less frequent urination may be a sign that inadequate amounts of fluids are being taken.

The water content of the body is partially controlled by the satisfaction of thirst, but sometimes thirst may lag behind the body's need. It's important to pay attention to your body's signals. When you thirst for water, by all means indulge yourself (unless your doctor has advised you to do otherwise). There's no danger that normal, healthy people will drink too much. Excess water will not accumulate in their bodies—it'll just be excreted. If the intake is too large, the urine that is produced will be more dilute.

You may have heard the terms "hard water" or "soft water." Hard water contains higher concentrations of calcium and magnesium than soft water . You can recognize hard water because it doesn't allow soap to lather easily. "Soft" water, which has a high sodium concentration, lathers easily.

It's been suggested that drinking large quantities of soft water adds a great deal of sodium to the diet and, in salt-sensitive people, may be responsible for the higher incidence of heart disease and high blood pressure in the areas of the country where soft water is prevalent. Bottled water may be hard or soft depending on its source.

Minerals in body fluids occur mainly as mineral salts. When these mineral salts dissolve in water, they may separate into ions—electrically charged particles called *electrolytes.* Sodium and potassium are the body's major electrolytes, and they're extremely im-

The Story of Minerals

portant. The movement of nutrients and wastes, respectively, into and out of cells is controlled primarily by the level and types of electrolytes.

Now, with a little background on minerals, you're ready to read the individual mineral profiles. When you've finished, you should have a better understanding of just how vital these inorganic elements really are in helping your body maintain good health.

Chapter 8
Mineral Profiles
Calcium

The main function of calcium is to build strong bones and teeth. As a matter of fact, 99 percent of all the calcium in the body is found within these structures. The remaining one percent is circulating in the blood or found in the body's soft tissues. However, this one percent plays many important roles. For example, it participates in blood clotting, muscle contraction and relaxation, transmission of nerve impulses, activation of enzymes, and hormone secretion.

Normally, a relationship exists between the amount of calcium in blood and the amount present in bones. The bones act as a reservoir of calcium, releasing it into the blood as it's needed.

Sources of Calcium

Milk, yogurt, cheese, and other dairy products are rich sources of calcium. Green vegetables, such as spinach, broccoli, kale, and chard, are also good sources. However, a small amount of the calcium in these vegetables may not be absorbed. This is due to the fact that they contain a substance called oxalic acid, which combines with calcium and prevents its absorption. This substance is found in chocolate as

Calcium

well. Even though the amount of calcium affected by the oxalic acid in these foods is extremely tiny, its been recommended by some experts that *chocolate milk* not be relied upon as a major source of calcium.

Phytic acid, a substance found in whole grains, also combines with calcium and other minerals, preventing their absorption. However, this only presents a problem in people who consume extremely large amounts of whole grains; in that case, a calcium supplement might be necessary to prevent a deficiency.

Recently, calcium compounds have been added to fruit juices and fruit drinks. This may eventually become an important source of this mineral. Mineral water, which has become a popular beverage, may also contribute some calcium to the diet, especially if it's used in large amounts.

Dietary Requirements for Calcium

The Recommended Dietary Allowance (RDA) for adults is 800 mg of calcium. For females who are pregnant or breast-feeding, the RDA is increased to 1,200 mg. One quart of milk contains approximately 1,000 mg of calcium. Two cups of milk or the equivalent (as described in the Basic Four Food Group guide in chapter 1) will contribute half of an adult's daily requirement for calcium. The rest of the calcium requirement can be obtained from foods like vegetables, breads, cereals, and dried peas and beans.

Calcium

Experts recommend that postmenopausal women get as much as 1,500 mg of calcium a day to help prevent or postpone osteoporosis. It's expected that when the RDA revision is published in the near future, the calcium recommendations may be increased for certain age groups.

Deficiency of Calcium

Deficiency of calcium can result in stunted growth and poor development of bones and teeth. A deficiency of this mineral, often caused by lack of vitamin D which is needed for calcium's normal absorption and use, is associated with a softening of bones. If you recall from your reading on vitamin D deficiency, this condition is referred to as rickets in children; osteomalacia in adults.

Osteoporosis, or adult bone loss, occurs in aging. If 1/3 or more of bone mass is lost, fractures may easily occur. One in four postmenopausal women develop osteoporosis; in men, the condition is less common. Low calcium intake during childhood and early onset of puberty appear to be important factors in the development of this condition.

Calcium Use and Misuse

When there's a deficiency of calcium, supplements are prescribed. Typically, these supplements also contain vitamin D to improve calcium absorption.

Continued on page 193

Calcium

Calcium Content of Foods

Food	Serving Size	Calcium* (mg)	Percent of U.S. RDA
Dairy Products			
Milk, whole	1 cup	285	29
Milk, skim	1 cup	296	30
Yogurt, low-fat	1 cup	350	35
Swiss cheese	1 ounce	270	27
American cheese	1 ounce	170	17
Cream cheese	1 ounce	23	2
Ice cream	1 cup	180	18
Meat, chicken, fish			
Salmon, pink, canned	4 ounces	220	22
Sardines, in oil	4 ounces	500	50
Chicken, roasted	½ pound	25	3
Hamburger with bun	4 ounces	75	8
Grains and breads			
Bread, enriched white	1 slice	26	3
Rice, white, cooked	1 cup	21	2
Bread, whole wheat	1 slice	20	2
Farina	1 cup	150	15
Fruits			
Apple	1	10	1
Figs, small dried	2	40	4
Vegetables			
Green beans	½ cup	63	6
Broccoli	1 cup	100	10
Kale	1 cup	160	16
Turnip greens	1 cup	250	25
Navy beans	1 cup	100	10

Calcium Content of Foods (continued)

Food	Serving Size	Calcium* (mg)	Percent of U.S. RDA
Vegetables			
Asparagus	½ cup	22	2
Cabbage, raw	1 cup	36	4
Nuts			
Almonds, roasted	1 ounce	67	7
Peanuts, roasted	1 ounce	20	2
Miscellaneous			
Tofu (bean curd)	4 ounces	150	15
Pretzels, thin	10	13	1
Soup, chicken noodle	¾ cup	24	2
Olives, green	10	24	2

*The U.S. RDA for calcium is 1,000 mg.

Continued from page 191

Recent research has indicated that calcium supplements may benefit some people who have high blood pressure. They may also be useful in preventing a condition that sometimes occurs in pregnancy called toxemia. In addition, research suggests that those people with higher intakes of calcium may be less likely to develop colon cancer. As a result of the publicity from these findings, *and* because many people don't get enough calcium in their diets, calcium supplements have become very popular.

Calcium

Calcium supplements may be used as an adjunct to estrogen-replacement therapy for the prevention of osteoporosis in postmenopausal women. However, the effectiveness of calcium supplementation for this purpose is still in question.

Calcium carbonate, which is 40 percent calcium, is one of the commonly used supplements. Crushed oyster shells or calcium-containing antacids contain this form of calcium. When you read the labels of calcium supplements, you should note that the milligrams in each tablet reflect both the calcium it contains, plus the carrier to which the calcium is bound. For example, the label may state "each tablet provides 1,250 mg of calcium carbonate, which yields 500 mg of elemental calcium." Some product labels may give the number of milligrams in a tablet and then give the percentage of the U. S. RDA for calcium that's supplied in each dose.

Large doses of calcium supplements—1,500 mg or more each day—may result in the formation of kidney stones in susceptible people. Most kidney stones are compounds of calcium oxylate.

Bone meal and dolomite have been suggested as "natural" sources of calcium, but since they may be contaminated with lead, arsenic, and other toxic metals, they are not recommended as safe supplements.

A number of calcium supplements are evaluated in the Vitamin and Mineral Supplement Profiles in the last chapter of this book.

Phosphorus

Phosphorus is essential for normal bone and teeth formation. It also participates in the further maintenance of bones throughout life. Phosphorus plays an important role in energy storage and release systems in the body. It's found in the genetic material, DNA (deoxyribonucleic acid) and RNA (ribonucleic acid), that represents the blueprints for the formation of new cells. In addition, phosphorus is necessary for normal milk secretion, and it participates in many metabolic reactions that occur in the body.

Good sources of phosphorus are milk and other dairy products, eggs, meat, fish, poultry, cheese, nuts, and whole grains. Even sodas and food additives supply some of this mineral.

The Recommended Dietary Allowance (RDA) for phosphorus is 800 mg a day for adults. For pregnant and nursing women, the RDA is increased to 1,200 mg. For most age groups, the RDA for phosphorus is the same as for calcium.

Although phosphorus deficiency has been reported in some infants fed cow's milk and in some people taking large amounts of antacids, a deficiency is unlikely. As a matter of fact, it's been estimated that

Continued on page 198

Phosphorus Content of Foods

Food	Serving Size	Phosphorus (mg)*	Percent of U.S. RDA
Dairy products			
Milk, whole	1 cup	227	23
Milk, skim	1 cup	233	23
Meat and equivalents			
Beef, rib roast	3 ounces	158	16
Frankfurter	1	76	8
Luncheon meat	¼ pound	189	19
Roast chicken, light meat	½ pound	617	62
Sardines, Atlantic, canned	3 ounces	424	42
Tuna, canned in water	3 ounces	199	20
Grains and breads			
Bread, enriched white	1 slice	28	3
Bread, whole wheat	1 slice	74	7
Rice, white, enriched, cooked	1 cup	57	6
Waffle	1	257	28
Fruits			
Grapefruit	1 medium	16	2
Apple	1	15	2
Figs dried	2 small	25	3
Vegetables			
Beans, green cooked	½ cup	46	5
Bean sprouts, cooked	1 cup	70	7
Broccoli	1 cup	101	10

Phosphorus Content of Foods (continued)

Food	Serving Size	Phosphorus (mg)*	Percent of U.S. RDA
Vegetables			
Cauliflower, cooked	1 cup	43	4
Corn, sweet, yellow, fresh	½ cup	75	8
Kidney beans, canned	1 cup	278	28
Lima beans, cooked	1 cup	293	29
Peppers, sweet, raw, green, chopped	½ cup	15	2
Pork and beans	1 cup	291	29
Potato, baked with skin	1	115	12
Nuts			
Almonds, roasted	1 ounce	143	14
Peanuts, roasted, salted	1 ounce	115	12
Butter	1 tablespoon	60	6
Pistachio nuts	1 ounce	143	14
Miscellaneous			
Shake, vanilla (10 oz.)	1	105	11
Soft drink	8 ounces	500	50
Pretzels, thin	10	79	8

*The U.S. RDA for phosphorus is 1,000 mg.

Phosphorus

Continued from page 195

some Americans may consume as much as four times their recommended dietary allowance.

Some nutrition experts believe that these excessive phosphorus intakes, when coupled with low intakes of calcium, may be a factor in the development of osteoporosis—adult bone loss. These experts feel that high levels of phosphorus can interfere with calcium absorption. They're concerned because the diets of some Americans are composed heavily of high-protein foods (such as meat, fish, or poultry), carbonated beverages or mineral-replacement drinks (commonly called sports drinks), and ready-to-eat convenience foods (which contain phosphate additives)—all of which may excessively increase the body's supply of phosphorus. These experts recommend, therefore, that phosphorus-rich foods or drinks (like any others) are consumed in moderation. They also feel that the ideal ratio of phosphorus to calcium in a particular food or drink is 1:1. For that reason, they consider milk a good source of phosphorus, since the quantities of phosphorus and calcium that it contains closely approach this ratio.

Magnesium

Although there's less than two ounces of magnesium in the body, it's a vital mineral. Magnesium is part of the mineral composition of bones and teeth. Actually, bones act as a reservoir of magnesium so that the mineral is available when needed. Magnesium plays a role in protein synthesis, muscle relaxation, and energy release. And it acts as a catalyst in important metabolic reactions.

Magnesium is found in most foods, especially green, leafy vegetables. This is because magnesium is part of chlorophyll, the pigment in plants that makes them green (and helps them trap sunlight for use in making food). Other good sources are dairy products, breads and cereals, nuts, chocolate, and dried peas and beans. Since magnesium is one of the minerals found in hard water, hard water is also a source.

The Recommended Dietary Allowance (RDA) for magnesium is 350 mg a day for men and 300 mg a day for women. Larger amounts are needed in women who are pregnant or breast-feeding.

Dietary deficiencies are unusual, but they can occur after prolonged vomiting, diarrhea, alcohol abuse,

Continued on page 201

Magnesium

Magnesium Content of Foods

Food	Serving Size	Magnesium (mg)*	Percent of U.S. RDA
Dairy products			
Milk, whole	1 cup	30	8
Yogurt, nonfat	1 cup	28	7
Cheddar cheese	1 ounce	8	2
Ice cream, vanilla, plain	½ cup	10	3
Eggs			
Whole, hard boiled	1 large	6	2
Grains and breads			
Bread, whole wheat	1 slice	26	7
Granola, ready-to-eat	½ cup	60	15
Oatmeal	½ cup	30	8
Noodles	⅔ cup	25	6
Rice, white, cooked	⅔ cup	10	3
Meat, fish, poultry			
Beef, chuck roast	3 oz.	20	5
Chicken, fried breast	½	10	3
Cod, steak, sauteed	4 oz.	30	8
Pork chop	1 medium	15	4
Lobster, Northern, meat	⅔ cup	20	5
Fruits			
Apple	1 medium	10	3
Avocado	½	55	14
Cherries, raw, sweet	10	10	3
Figs, dried	5	56	14

Magnesium Content of Foods (continued)

Food	Serving Size	Magnesium (mg)*	Percent of U.S. RDA
Fruits			
Plum, raw	1 medium	6	2
Strawberries, whole, fresh	⅔ cup	12	3
Vegetables			
Asparagus, fresh	½ cup	15	4
Beans, lima, boiled	½ cup	55	14
Blackeyed peas, cooked	1 cup	117	29
Broccoli, cooked	1 cup	94	24
Cauliflower, cooked	½ cup	8	2
Garbanzo beans, cooked	1 cup	117	29
Mushrooms, raw	½ cup	5	1

*The U.S. RDA for magnesium is 400 mg.

Continued from page 199

or long-term use of diuretics (water pills). A magnesium deficiency may also occur if a person has a severe protein deficiency. High intakes of calcium can increase the excretion of magnesium and can lead to problems if unchecked.

Magnesium

Magnesium deficiency can lead to a loss of muscle control by causing muscles to remain contracted. Nervousness, irritability, and tremors are other symptoms. A deficiency of magnesium may be the cause of hallucinations in people who are undergoing alcohol withdrawal.

Research indicates that people who regularly drink hard water that's high in magnesium have a lower incidence of sudden death from heart failure than do people who regularly drink soft water. It has been suggested that magnesium intake may be a factor in lowering blood pressure. For example, magnesium supplements have been shown to lower blood pressure in people taking diuretics (water pills). Magnesium compounds have also been used to treat high blood pressure in pregnant women. However, more research is needed to determine the significance of magnesium's role, if any, in the regulation of blood pressure.

Chlorine

Chlorine plays a role in various systems of internal regulation including water balance, acid-base balance, and osmotic pressure. For example, it's part of the hydrochloric acid of the stomach that's needed for normal digestion. Maintaining a certain level of acidity in the stomach is also necessary to ensure proper absorption of food, as well as to reduce the growth of harmful bacteria.

Regular table salt is 60 percent chlorine (in the form of chloride). This source, along with salt that occurs naturally in foods, provides all the chlorine needed. There is no Recommended Dietary Allowance (RDA) for chlorine. Instead there's a suggested safe and adequate range of intake of 1,700 to 5,100 mg a day for adults.

A chlorine deficiency is not likely because it can be acquired from so many sources, but it *can* happen under certain circumstances. For example, several years ago, some infant formula was prepared without any chlorine. Children fed this formula as their sole source of food did develop chlorine deficiencies.

Sodium

Function of Sodium

In the body, sodium plays a major role in regulating water balance. It's also important in maintaining the body's ability to regulate acid-base balance, transmit nerve impulses, regulate cell membrane function and muscle activity, and absorb and transport certain nutrients. Sodium is also part of body substances like sweat and tears.

Sources of Sodium

Sodium is found in most foods either naturally or as an additive in processing or preparation. Celery, carrots, greens, beets, eggs, or milk, for example, are naturally high in sodium. Foods like sour pickles, luncheon meats, canned vegetables, soups, and frozen dinners, on the other hand, often have sodium or salt (sodium chloride) added during processing.

You can't always tell by the taste if a food is high in sodium. For example, ice cream and prepared puddings are often high in sodium, even though they don't usually taste salty. Some foods are naturally low in sodium, like fruits, rice, pasta, and oatmeal and other grains.

Even substances such as toothpaste and mouthwash contain sodium. So does the drinking water in many areas.

Since July 1986, the sodium content of foods must be included as part of a nutrition label. Terms that the manufacturer may use to describe the sodium content per serving are defined as follows:

- sodium free—less than 5 mg per serving
- very low sodium—35 mg or less per serving
- low sodium—140 mg or less per serving
- reduced sodium—processed to reduce the usual level of sodium by 75 percent
- unsalted—processed without the form of salt normally used (table salt)
- low salt—made with less salt than the usual variety of the same food

Dietary Requirements of Sodium

Americans eat about five to seven grams (5,000 to 7,000 mg) of sodium a day. This amount is derived mainly from sodium chloride—common table salt. About 40 percent of this compound is sodium. It's estimated that a daily intake of only 500 mg of sodium would meet the body's actual need for this mineral.

Continued on page 207

Sodium

Sodium Content of Common Foods

Food	Serving Size	Milligrams of Sodium*
Cheddar cheese	1 ounce	168
Ice cream, 10% fat	1 cup	84
Milk, whole	1 cup	122
Egg, whole, large	1	61
Butter or margarine	1 tablespoon	140
Beef, ground	1 cup	55
Chicken, fried	1¾ ounces	34
Pork, roasted	4½ ounces	74
Turkey	3 ounces	111
Apples	1	1
Juice, cranberry cocktail	1 cup	3
Raisins, seedless	1 cup	39
Bread, white	1 slice	142
Beans, dry	1 cup	34
Peanut butter	1 tablespoon	97
Jam or preserves	1 tablespoon	2
Asparagus, cooked	1 cup	1
Potato, baked, no skin	1	6
Zucchini, cooked	1 cup	2
Brewer's yeast, dried	1 tablespoon	10
Baking powder, sodium aluminum sulfate	1 tablespoon	1,205
Soy sauce	1 fluid ounce	2,666
Potato chips	14	133
Sauerkraut	1 cup	1,561
Pickle, dill	1	928
Olives, green	10	936
Tomato juice	1 cup	881

*There is no U.S. RDA for sodium. The *safe and adequate daily intake* is 1,100 to 3,300 mg.

Continued from page 205

Even though there's no Recommended Dietary Allowance (RDA) for sodium, *there is a suggested safe and adequate range of intake:* 1,100 to 3,300 mg a day.

Deficiency of Sodium

Since the body has a large reserve of sodium, and since under normal circumstances people are continuously eating sodium-containing foods, a deficiency is not likely. However, *salt* depletion can temporarily occur through profuse sweating, if strenuous, prolonged activity is undertaken in warm weather or hot climates. Even in this situation, salt that's been lost can be easily replaced by eating salty foods.

Sodium Use and Misuse

Supplements of sodium chloride are not commonly recommended for general use, so this section will deal with dietary salt intake.

Studies have shown that a relationship may exist between salt intake and the incidence of hypertension—a condition commonly called high blood pressure. It's been noted that high blood pressure rarely appears in cultures with low salt intakes. Researchers suspect that high salt intakes over extended periods of time may contribute to this condition. However, it also appears that some people may be more sus-

Sodium

ceptible than others to developing high blood pressure. Because of this, a person with a family history of hypertension may be advised by his or her doctor to eat a low-salt diet and have regular blood pressure check-ups.

Since Americans as a group have a rather large salt intake, and since the incidence of high blood pressure increases as people age, a low-salt diet might actually be a wise choice for everyone (unless otherwise directed by a doctor).

People who already have high blood pressure are generally advised to reduce their salt intake. However, research indicates that only about half of those people—those who are salt sensitive—will benefit by salt restriction.

Potassium

The body normally contains about nine grams of potassium. Most of it is found inside body cells. Potassium plays an important role in maintaining water balance and acid-base balance. It participates in the transmission of nerve impulses and in the transfer of messages from nerves to muscles. It also acts as a catalyst in carbohydrate and protein metabolism.

Because potassium is a constant part of lean body mass (muscle), measurements of potassium content may be used to estimate body composition in research studies.

Studies suggest that a high intake of potassium-rich foods may reduce blood pressure and the risk of stroke. Theoretically, when potassium intake is high, more sodium is excreted from the body and blood pressure is lowered. Vegetarians, for example, are known to have lower blood pressure values than their nonvegetarian counterparts. Their high potassium intakes from the large amounts of fruits and vegetables they consume may be a factor.

Some diuretics (water pills) commonly used to treat high blood pressure cause potassium to be lost from

Continued on page 211

Potassium Content of Foods

Food	Serving Size	Milligrams of Potassium*
Dairy products		
Yogurt	1 cup	406
Milk, whole	1 cup	370
Cheddar cheese	1 ounce	28
Breads and cereals		
Brewer's yeast	1 tablespoon	152
Wheat bran	¼ cup	103
Whole-wheat bread	1 slice	50
Beans, peas, nuts		
Lima beans, cooked	1 cup	1,163
Pinto beans, cooked	1 cup	882
Kidney beans, canned	1 cup	673
Peas, split, cooked	1 cup	592
Peanuts, dried, unsalted	1 ounce	204
Meat, fish, poultry		
Sirloin steak, lean	8 ounces	928
Sole/flounder, baked	3 ounces	272
Chicken breast, roasted	½	220
Fruits		
Cantaloupe melon	½	825
Watermelon	1 slice	560
Orange juice	1 cup	496
Banana	1	451
Apricots	3	313
Orange	1	237
Peach	1	171
Apple	1	159

Potassium Content of Foods (continued)

Food	Serving Size	Milligrams of Potassium*
Vegetables		
Winter squash, baked	1 cup	1,071
Potato, baked, with skin	1	844
Spinach, cooked	1 cup	834
Bok choy, cooked	1 cup	630
Asparagus	1 cup	558
Beets, cooked	1 cup	532
Zucchini, cooked	1 cup	455
Cauliflower	1 cup	400
Broccoli	1 cup	254
Romaine lettuce	1 cup	162
Celery	1 stalk	114
Red radishes	10	104

*There is no U.S. RDA for potassium. The *safe and adequate daily intake* is 1,875 to 5,625 mg.

Continued from page 209

the body. To compensate, people being treated with these types of diuretics are generally advised to eat foods that are rich in potassium. Milk, meat, tomatoes, prunes, bananas, oranges, and dried peas and beans are good sources of potassium. Most unprocessed, whole foods contain potassium. Many salt substitutes are compounds of potassium chloride and can be a source of potassium in the diet.

Potassium

Because potassium is found in so many foods, a dietary deficiency is unlikely. However, uncontrolled diabetes or a long period of excessive water loss (as from sweating) may result in potassium depletion. Muscle weakness can be an early sign that potassium depletion is occurring.

A typical American diet is estimated to provide about two to five grams of potassium daily. There is no Recommended Dietary Allowance (RDA) for potassium, but there is *an estimated safe and adequate range of intake*: 1,875 to 5,625 mg a day for adults.

Under normal circumstances, potassium supplements are not recommended for general use. They are prescribed only in specific instances. For example, they may be prescribed for people who are taking certain types of diuretics in order to prevent depletion.

Sulfur

Sulfur is found throughout the body, especially in the skin, hair, and nails. Sulfur is involved in the storage and release of energy. It's part of the genetic material of cells, and helps promote enzyme reactions and blood clotting. Sulfur also combines with certain toxic materials that enter the body so they can be passed out safely in the urine.

There is no Recommended Dietary Allowance for sulfur. It's been found that when protein intake is adequate, sulfur intake is adequate as well. This is because sulfur-containing amino acids (the building blocks of protein) supply the body with the amount of sulfur it needs. Sulfur is also part of two B vitamins—biotin and thiamin.

Cheese, eggs, fish, poultry, grains, nuts, and dried peas and beans are rich sources of sulfur.

Iron

Function of Iron

The body contains only three to five grams of iron, an amount approximately equal to a teaspoon. Most of this is found in the hemoglobin of red blood cells—the pigment that gives these blood cells their red color. Hemoglobin transports oxygen and carbon dioxide respectively to and from the cells of the body. Iron is also an essential element in the chain of enzyme-controlled reactions that release energy.

Sources of Iron

Good sources of iron include liver and other meats, whole grains, shellfish, green leafy vegetables, and nuts. Iron is one of the nutrients added to enriched cereals and bread. Recently soybean hulls (not the whole soybean) were shown to contain a very absorbable form of iron. In the future, these hulls will probably be used to fortify other foods with iron. It's important to note that milk is a poor source of iron and should not be relied on as such, especially in the diets of infants and children.

Iron

Cooking in iron pots adds iron to the foods prepared in them. This is especially true if these foods are acidic, such as tomatoes. Even eggs fried in iron skillets pick up some of the iron from the pan.

Dietary Requirements for Iron

The Recommended Dietary Allowance (RDA) for iron is 10 mg for adult males and postmenopausal females, and 18 mg for menstruating females. The RDA for iron is increased for both pregnant and breast-feeding women. Iron requirements are also greater during periods of growth and development.

Deficiency of Iron

It's estimated that the typical American diet provides 6 mg of iron in every 1,000 calories taken in. Because many women take in fewer than 2,000 calories a day, their diets may actally provide less than 12 mg of iron. From these figures, it becomes obvious that many women may not acquire enough iron to meet their recommended dietary allowances. Men, on the other hand, who may eat 2,500 calories a day or more, are more likely to get their recommended iron intakes.

Only about 10 percent of the iron in foods is absorbed. The iron in meat, called heme iron, is absorbed better than the non-heme iron found in vegetables. The soy hulls mentioned earlier are an exception.

Continued on page 217

Iron Content of Foods

Food	Amount	Iron (mg)*	Percent of U.S. RDA
Meat, fish, poultry			
Liver, calf or lamb	2 slices	13.4	74
Liver, beef or chicken	¼-½ cup	5.0	28
Beef, lamb, pork, veal; cooked	3 ounces	2.5	14
Fish	3 ounces	1.0	6
Chicken breast	1 whole	1.8	10
Grains and breads			
Bread, enriched or whole grain	3 slices	1.7	10
Cereals, enriched, ready-to-eat	1 ounce	1.3	9
Spaghetti, noodles, macaroni, cooked	3 ounces	1.0	6
Vegetables			
Spinach, cooked	½ cup	2.0	12
Beet greens, cooked	½ cup	1.9	11
Potato, white	1 medium	0.7	4
Soybeans, cooked	½ cup	2.5	14
Beans, lima, cooked	½ cup	2.0	11
Peas, green, cooked	½ cup	1.4	7
Fruits			
Figs, dried	2 small	0.9	5
Raisins	2 tablespoons	0.6	3
Peach, raw	1 medium	0.6	3
Grapes	22-24 average	0.4	2
Cherries	20-25 small	0.4	2

*The U.S. RDA for iron is 18 mg.

Continued from page 215

Meat, fish, poultry, and vitamin C all increase iron absorption. Having any of these foods at a meal will also increase the amount of iron absorbed from other foods eaten during that meal. Coffee, tea, whole soybeans, and whole grains, on the other hand, will all reduce the amount of iron absorbed from foods eaten at the same meal.

Iron deficiency can cause the most common type of anemia—iron deficiency anemia. Headache, shortness of breath, weakness, fatigue, heart palpitations, and sore tongue are some of the symptoms. For people who are anemic, even mild exercise can cause chest pain. Mild iron deficiency even without anemia has been shown to cause learning problems in school children.

Pica, an abnormal desire to eat nonfood substances like clay, chalk, ashes, or laundry starch (none of which contain iron) is sometimes seen along with iron deficiency. That's because the eating of such nonfoods (clay, for example) may interfere with iron absorption and may be a factor contributing to the anemia.

Continued use of aspirin can cause bleeding in the lining of the stomach and may lead to iron deficiency because of blood loss.

Young children who are given excessively large amounts of milk and few other foods have been shown to develop a milk-induced anemia. As we said before, the milk contains little iron, and in very

Iron

large quantities may actually promote irritation and bleeding in the stomach.

The normal acidity of the stomach helps promote iron absorption in the intestine. By reducing the acidity of the stomach, such as with the chronic use of antacids, the amount of iron absorbed is also reduced, and a deficiency may result.

It's estimated that 8 percent of the women and one percent of the men in the United States have symptoms of iron deficiency. It's estimated that even larger numbers of people have inadequate iron reserves. This is probably due to poor food choices or the lack of adequate food intake. Despite these statistics, the incidence of iron deficiency anemia in the infants and preschool children of low-income families has actually been declining. In 1975, it was 7.7 percent. In 1985, it was 2.9 percent. The improved iron status is believed due, at least in part, to the fact that the Special Supplemental Food Program for Women, Infants, and Children (WIC) supplies iron-fortified formula to bottle-fed infants.

Iron Use and Misuse

Iron supplements, along with an iron-rich diet, are useful in treating iron deficiency. Iron is available in both a *ferrous* and *ferric* form. Iron in the ferrous form is better absorbed than ferric iron. And, it appears that all ferrous salts of iron are absorbed equally well. When you read labels of iron supplements, you should note that the milligrams of each tablet reflects both the iron it contains, plus the carrier to which it's bound. For example, the label may state "each tablet provides 200 mg of ferrous fumarate, which yields 67 mg of elemental iron."

Some people don't tolerate iron supplements well and may develop such side effects as heartburn, nausea, stomachache, constipation, or diarrhea. Taking the supplement along with food and gradually working up to the desired dose (instead of starting with a high dose) may avoid or minimize these symptoms. Since part of the iron is not absorbed, the stool may become dark.

It's estimated that iron poisoning is the second most common type of accidental poisoning in young children. (Aspirin is the most common.) Iron tablets are often coated with sugar to mask their unpleasant taste, and if allowed access to them, children may eat them like candy. *EXCESS IRON INTAKE CAN BE FATAL. All supplements should be kept out of the reach of children.*

In normal, healthy people, the intestine controls the amount of iron that's absorbed. If iron reserves have been depleted, the rate of absorption is greatly accelerated. When the body has become saturated with iron, the rate of iron absorption from the intestinal tract greatly decreases. If, for some reason, the intestine does not, or cannot, properly perform this function, the results can be toxic.

For example, a certain percent of the population suffers from hemochromatosis, a hereditary disease, in

Iron

which too much iron is absorbed and deposited in body tissues. The symptoms of this condition include weakness, weight loss, change in skin color, abdominal pain, loss of the desire for sex, and the onset of diabetes. When examined, heart, liver, or joint impairment may also be found. The treatment for this disease involves the removal of excess body iron, in addition to supportive treatment of damaged organs.

High intakes of alcohol over extended periods of time can damage the intestine so that too much iron is absorbed. Some alcoholic drinks, particularly red wine, even contain substantial amounts of iron that can add to the overload. It's important to remember that prolonged excessive absorption of iron can be highly dangerous.

Iodine

Function of Iodine

Of the 25 mg of iodine in the body, almost half is found in the thyroid gland. Iodine is an important component of thyroid hormones—the hormones that control energy metabolism in the body. Normal body temperature, basal metabolic rate, reproduction, and growth all depend on these vital hormones.

Sources of Iodine

Seafood is a good source of iodine. Iodized salt, which has been in use since 1924, is another rich source. One teaspoon of iodized salt provides 260 µg (micrograms) of iodine, nearly twice the RDA. The amount of iodine in vegetables and grains depends on the amount of iodine that was present in the soil in which they were grown. In certain regions of the world, this amount is less than optimal.

Iodine-containing compounds are used to disinfect dairy equipment, and iodine-containing feed is fed to dairy cattle. Both of these sources contribute to the amount of iodine in our milk and dairy products.

Iodine

Iodine may also be found in dough conditioners used by bakeries, in food colorings, and even in polluted air.

Dietary Requirements for Iodine

The Recommended Dietary Allowance (RDA) for adults is 150 µg a day. It's estimated that the average intake in the United States is about four times that amount.

Deficiency of Iodine

A deficiency of iodine causes the thyroid gland to enlarge beyond its normal size. The thyroid gland, which is normally about the size of a lima bean, can become as large as a person's head! A deficiency of thyroid hormones may result in such symptoms as mental and physical sluggishness, slowed heart rate, weight gain, constipation, and increased sleeping time (14-16 hours per day). In pregnancy, the results of iodine deficiency may have even more serious repercussions. The baby of an iodine-deficient mother may have retarded physical and mental development—a condition known as cretinism.

Certain substances known as goitrogens may induce goiter when iodine intake is low. Cabbage, brussels sprouts, rutabagas, cauliflower, turnips, and peanuts contain these substances. However, since heat destroys goitrogens, the potential dangers associated with them should only exist if large amounts of these foods are eaten raw.

Iodine Use and Misuse

In view of the fact that Americans are taking in several times the RDA for iodine, iodine supplements are rarely needed. In fact, some experts are even questioning the value of iodizing table salt, since they feel it may not actually be necessary.

Some people who are overweight because of overeating and underexercising mistakenly blame their overweight condition on an underactive thyroid gland. In the hopes of speeding up their metabolism, they may take excess iodine in supplement form or in the form of sea salt or various seaweeds like kelp. In very large amounts, iodine can be poisonous.

Some people are sensitive to this mineral and may break out in a rash if their iodine intake is excessively large. The rash looks somewhat like acne, but will disappear when excess iodine intake is reduced. During certain x-ray procedures, such as urography (x ray of the kidneys), a form of iodine may be used in the injectable contrast medium—the substance which allows an organ or body part to be visualized on x-ray film. If a person is allergic to iodine, a rash may occur following injection of the material.

Zinc

Function of Zinc

The majority of the 2 to 3 grams of zinc in the body is found within the bones. The rest of this trace mineral is found mostly in the skin, hair, and nails. It's been estimated that the prostate gland of the male contains more zinc than any other organ. Zinc is part of over 70 different enzyme systems that function in the metabolism of carbohydrates, fats, and proteins. Zinc is part of the hormone insulin (a hormone that helps regulate blood sugar levels), and plays an important role in the transport of vitamin A from its storage in the liver so that it can be used in the body.

Sources of Zinc

Oysters have more zinc than any other food. Meat, poultry, eggs, and liver are also rich sources. It's estimated that two servings of animal protein daily will provide most of the zinc needed by a healthy person. Whole grains contain fair amounts of zinc, but they also contain phytates, substances that combine with the zinc and prevent its absorption. Yeast counteracts the action of phytates, so when eating whole grain breads, for example, a yeast-containing selection may be a wise choice.

Dietary Requirements for Zinc

The Recommended Dietary Allowance (RDA) for zinc is 15 mg daily, with larger amounts recommended during pregnancy and breast-feeding. Experts estimate that the average American diet provides about 10 mg a day.

Deficiency of Zinc

Severe deficiency of zinc, as is found among certain populations of underdeveloped countries, has serious effects. It retards growth and sexual development, delays healing of wounds, causes a low sperm count, depresses the body's immune system (making infections more likely), and reduces appetite. Zinc depletion causes reduced taste and smell sensations.

Low zinc intakes may be a factor in a condition that sometimes occurs in pregnancy called toxemia and may also contribute to a decreased birth weight of the baby. (Low-birthweight babies are generally at greater risk of health problems than babies of normal weight.)

Although there's little data to support this idea at the present time, it's suspected that marginal zinc intakes are common in the United States. Studies in

Continued on page 227

Zinc Content of Foods

Food	Amount	Zinc (mg)*	Percent of U.S. RDA
Dairy products			
Milk, whole	1 cup	1.0	15
American cheese	1 ounce	0.8	5
Egg, whole	1 large	0.7	5
Cereals and breads			
Bread, white, enriched	1 slice	0.2	1
Bran flakes, ready-to-eat	1 cup	1.3	9
Grains			
Rice, brown	⅔ cup	0.8	5
Noodles, enriched, cooked	½ cup	0.6	4
Beans, peas, nuts			
Soybeans, cooked	½ cup	0.6	4
Peas, split, cooked	½ cup	1.1	7
Peanut butter	1 tablespoon	0.4	3
Meat, fish, poultry			
Beef, chuck	3 ounces	3.7	25
Chicken, light meat, no skin	3 ounces	0.9	6
Salmon, steak, broiled	1	2.4	16
Oysters, Eastern, raw	6	90.0	600
Fruits			
Orange	1	0.3	2
Pineapple	1 cup	0.3	2

Zinc Content of Foods (continued)

Food	Amount	Zinc (mg)*	Percent of U.S. RDA
Vegetables			
Broccoli, cooked	½ cup	0.2	1
Carrot, raw	1	0.3	2
Tomato, raw	1	0.3	2
Potato, baked	1	0.4	3

*The U.S. RDA for zinc is 15 mg.

Continued from page 225

the elderly have shown that as many as 90 percent have intakes of zinc below the RDA. The decreased consumption of meat, which has become a fairly common health practice in the American diet, results in reduced zinc intake. Low-calorie diets, which are also popular, may be low in zinc as well.

Vegetarian diets, especially those that do not contain any animal products, are likely to result in zinc deficiency. Vegetarians should be encouraged to eat whole-grain breads that are made with yeast. The yeast breaks down the phytates in the whole grains so that the zinc can be absorbed better. In unleavened bread like pita and flat bread, the phytates are intact and can tie up the zinc so that it's not absorbed. Strict vegetarians should consult their doctors about the use of a zinc supplement of about 15 mg a day to prevent deficiency. Because zinc absorption

Zinc

is reduced by the presence of iron, the zinc component of multimineral supplements containing iron may not be well absorbed. It's best to take a zinc supplement by itself, on an empty stomach (unless otherwise advised by a doctor).

Infections, injuries, or other physical sources of stress, can cause excess zinc to be lost in the urine. Pica, the eating of nonfood substances such as clay, chalk, ashes, or laundry starch, can reduce the amount of zinc absorbed. If a deficiency of zinc is diagnosed, zinc supplements may be beneficial.

Zinc Use and Misuse

Zinc is a popular supplement. Many people suffer from loss of smell and taste due to aging, treatment for cancer, or serious infections. In some people, zinc supplements have been found to be useful in restoring these sensations.

Zinc is also given to improve healing in people with bedsores and other wounds. In these situations, however, zinc supplements are probably only useful if the patients are deficient in the mineral. Zinc supplements have also been suggested to help reduce perspiration odor and treat acne. The effectiveness of this treatment is still in question.

It's been found that people with sickle cell anemia may lose a lot of zinc in their urine. Use of zinc supplements can be helpful in preventing deficiency.

Zinc absorption is reduced in a rare inherited disease called acrodermatitis enteropathica. Symptoms, which include eczema, hair loss, retarded growth, and emotional problems, can be controlled by zinc supplementation.

Zinc has also been used successfully to treat the abnormally large copper accumulations that occur in people who suffer from a rare inherited disorder called Wilson's disease.

Excess zinc supplementation in amounts greater than 50 mg a day can cause copper deficiency and anemia. Intakes of large amounts of zinc can cause vomiting, diarrhea, fever, kidney failure, and even death. This type of poisoning has actually occurred in the past, when certain foods and drinks were contaminated by galvanized containers, whose zinc coatings leached into their contents.

Fluoride

Function of Fluoride

Fluoride is an essential trace mineral found in bones, teeth, and body fluids. If fluoride is available during the development of bones and teeth, it's incorporated into their structure, making the teeth more resistant to decay and the bones more resistant to osteoporosis (adult bone loss). Fluoride also maintains the structure of bones and teeth after they're formed.

Studies indicate that children raised in areas where there is one part per million of fluoride in the water have 50 percent less cavities than children who do not drink fluoridated water.

Sources of Fluoride

Water is the usual source of fluoride in the diet. Fish and tea are good sources of fluoride as well. It's estimated that there's an average of 0.2 mg of fluoride in a cup of tea.

Dietary Requirements for Fluoride

There is no Recommended Dietary Allowance (RDA) for fluoride, but there is a *suggested safe and adequate range of intake* of 1.5 to 4.0 mg daily.

Deficiency of Fluoride

Research has shown that people who live in areas where the drinking water contains less than one part per million of fluoride have an increased incidence of dental decay and osteoporosis (adult bone loss).

Fluoride Use and Misuse

In many areas of the country, fluoride is added to the drinking water at a level of one part per million which is the optimum level. In some communities where the natural fluoride concentration in the water is high (2 to 8 parts per million) children's teeth develop with mottled (spotted) enamel—a condition called fluorosis. This condition doesn't seem to be harmful; in fact, mottled teeth are very resistant to decay. However, they don't have the "healthy," sparkling white appearance that the media promotes so heavily.

In some areas, there is strong opposition to adding fluoride to the drinking water. Opponents claim that fluoridated water increases the incidence of cancer and birth defects, and causes other health problems.

Fluoride

However, there's no established evidence that drinking water containing one part per million of fluoride is harmful. In fact, fluoridation may well be one of the most thoroughly studied community health measures in recent history. The U.S. Public Health Service, state and local health departments, the World Health Organization (WHO), the National Cancer Institute, and the U.S. Center for Disease Control are among the agencies that have unanimously refuted any claims linking fluoridation to public health risks. The only sign of physical change in life-long users of optimally fluoridated water is a decreased incidence of tooth decay and osteoporosis.

Copper

There's about 75 to 100 mg of copper in the body. Copper helps the body absorb and use iron. It's part of several enzymes that help form hemoglobin (the oxygen-carrying pigment in red blood cells) and collagen (a connective tissue protein).

Sources of copper include shellfish, liver, dried peas and beans, nuts, cocoa, fruits, and vegetables. There's no Recommended Dietary Allowance (RDA) for copper, but there's a *suggested safe and adequate range of intake* of 2.0 to 3.0 mg. It's estimated that the average American diet provides about 2.0 mg.

A deficiency of copper is very rare, but it has been found in severely malnourished children whose growth and metabolism were disturbed.

Excess intake, which has been reported to occur after drinking water that was stored in copper tanks, causes headache, dizziness, and vomiting.

A rare, inherited disorder called Wilson's disease causes abnormally high accumulations of copper in the body. It's treated with certain medications and/or zinc supplements.

Chromium

Chromium is part of the glucose tolerance factor (GTF), which regulates the metabolism of glucose in the body. GTF increases the action of insulin, a hormone involved in glucose metabolism. (Glucose is the form in which sugar and starch are used by the body). When there's a lack of chromium, insulin doesn't function properly. Chromium supplements can improve the body's ability to handle glucose, but only if there's a chromium deficiency.

Chromium is found in whole grains, meats, cheese, eggs, and yeast. More refined foods contain less chromium. There is no Recommended Dietary Allowance (RDA) for chromium. However, there's a *suggested safe and adequate range of intake* of 0.05 to 0.2 mg. Experts caution us not to exceed this intake on a daily basis.

Manganese

There's about 20 mg of manganese in the body. Manganese is involved in bone formation and growth of connective tissue, and is an activator of many enzymes that function in metabolism.

Good sources are nuts, whole grains, and dried peas and beans. There's no Recommended Dietary Allowance (RDA) for manganese. However, there's a *suggested safe and adequate range of intake* of 2.5 to 5.0 mg a day. Deficiencies have not been reported.

Miners who have been exposed to large amounts of manganese dust over long periods of time have shown symptoms of brain disease.

Selenium

Selenium is found in all body tissues, with the highest concentrations in the kidneys, liver, spleen, pancreas, and testicles. Selenium functions with vitamin E as an antioxidant (a substance that prevents oxidation), helping to prevent cell damage that may occur from the breakdown products of fats.

Severe deficiency of selenium affects heart function. Deficiencies are hard to detect because vitamin E can substitute for selenium in some of its functions.

Meat and fish are rich sources of selenium. The amount found in grains depends upon the level of the mineral found in the soil in which they were grown. There is no Recommended Dietary Allowance (RDA) for selenium. However, there's a *suggested safe and adequate range of intake* of 0.05 to 0.2 mg. A typical American diet generally provides this amount.

Some studies suggest that selenium *may have* anti-cancer properties. This suggestion is based on the fact that cancer rates are high in areas of the world where the soil contains little selenium. However, a great deal more research is necessary to determine selenium's role (if any) in reducing the risk of cancer.

Too much selenium can be poisonous. If selenium supplements are taken, they should contain no more than the estimated safe range noted earlier in this chapter.

Selenium Content of Common Foods

Food	Serving Size	Selenium (μg)*
Meat loaf	3½ ounces	17
Liver, beef	3½ ounces	56
Bacon	1 ounce	7
Frankfurter	1	5
Salmon, canned	3½ ounces	75
Tuna, canned	3½ ounces	72
Egg	1	7
Peanut butter	1 ounce	2.5
Milk, skim	1 cup	6
Milk, whole	1 cup	6
Bagel	1	20
Cornflakes	1¼ cup	2
Granola	¾ cup	19
Bread, white	1 slice	8
Bread, cracked wheat	1 slice	17
Noodles, egg	⅔ cup	19
Waffle	1	13
Cucumber	1 ounce	2
Orange	1	2
Chicken rice soup	1 cup	3
Codfish	3½ ounces	45
Crab, canned	3½ ounces	22

*There is no U.S. RDA for selenium. The *safe and adequate daily intake* is 50 to 200 μg.

Molybdenum

There's only about 9 mg of molybdenum in the body. It functions as part of the enzyme systems involved in the metabolism of carbohydrates, fats and proteins.

Good sources of molybdenum are liver, wheat germ, whole grains, and dried peas and beans. The molybdenum content of food varies according to the level that was present in the soil from which it came.

There's no Recommended Dietary Allowance (RDA), but there is a *suggested safe and adequate range of intake* of 0.15 to 0.50 mg daily. That amount is easily acquired in the average diet.

There have been reports of toxic effects associated with excess intakes of molybdenum. Some reports have shown that gout-like symptoms may occur. Supplements of this mineral should not be taken (unless otherwise directed by a doctor).

Cobalt

As part of vitamin B_{12}, cobalt plays a major role in the body's metabolic processes. There's no Recommended Dietary Allowance (RDA) for cobalt since the amount needed is acquired as part of vitamin B_{12}.

Other Trace Minerals

Nickel, silicon, tin, and vanadium are other trace minerals that, at the present time, are not considered essential elements for humans. However, since studies show that they may be necessary for animals, the possibility exists that at some time in the future, these minerals may be found to be important for us as well.

Chapter 9

Supplement Product Profiles

Although it has been our contention throughout this book that there's no substitute for a healthy diet, we also know that nutrition needs can change with time and circumstance. In light of this, we've profiled over 100 of the vitamin, mineral, and vitamin/mineral products most commonly used in this country so that you know what kinds of supplements are available. In each profile, you will find the product name, the manufacturer, the dosage form (e.g. capsules, tablets), and the types and amounts of ingredients contained within. Other information, such as warnings or possible side effects, is included as it applies.

CONSUMER GUIDE® does not recommend the use of supplements by people who are in good health and eat a balanced diet. However, if you're in doubt as to your vitamin and/or mineral status, check with your doctor. After a thorough evaluation of your diet, eating habits, state of health, and other factors that may affect your current nutrition needs, he or she can help you determine whether supplements are necessary, and if they are, which ones might be beneficial.

ALBEE C-800 PLUS IRON
(multivitamin supplement with iron)

Manufacturer: A.H. Robins Company
Dosage form: Tablets
Ingredients:

vitamin C	800 mg
thiamin (B_1)	15 mg
riboflavin (B_2)	17 mg
niacin	100 mg
vitamin B_6	25 mg
pantothenic acid	25 mg
vitamin E	45 IU
folic acid	0.4 mg
vitamin B_{12}	12 µg
iron	27 mg

Comments:

- This product contains greater than 100 percent of the U.S. RDA for all nutrients except folic acid.
- Vitamin C, B_1, and B_2 are provided in megadose amounts (ten or more times the U.S. RDA).
- Accidental iron poisoning is a real possiblity, especially with young children. *Be sure all nutrient supplements are stored out of their reach.*
- Iron interacts with oral tetracycline antibiotics, reducing their absorption.
- Consult your pharmacist or physician for further information.

Supplement Product Profiles

BETA-CAROTENE (vitamin supplement)

Manufacturer: Nature's Bounty, Inc.
Dosage form: Capsules
Ingredients:

Beta-carotene (provitamin A)   25,000 IU

Comments: There is no RDA recommendation for beta-carotene. Ample provitamin A is provided by selection of beta-carotene-rich deep yellow or dark orange vegetables and fruits, and green, leafy vegetables.

BUGS BUNNY CHILDREN'S CHEWABLE VITAMINS + MINERALS
(multivitamin/mineral supplement)

Manufacturer: Miles Laboratories, Inc.
Dosage form: Chewable tablets
Nutrients:

vitamin A	5,000 IU
vitamin D	400 IU
vitamin E	30 IU
vitamin C	60 mg
folic acid	0.4 mg
thiamin (B_1)	1.5 mg
riboflavin (B_2)	1.7 mg
niacin	20 mg
vitamin B_6	2 mg
vitamin B_{12}	6 μg
biotin	40 μg
pantothenic acid	10 mg

iron	18 mg
calcium	100 mg
copper	2 mg
phosphorus	100 mg
iodine	150 μg
magnesium	20 mg
zinc	15 mg

Comments:

- This product is sugar free.
- Accidental iron poisoning is a real possibility, especially with young children. *Be sure all nutrient supplements are stored out of their reach.*
- Iron interacts with oral tetracycline antibiotics, reducing their absorption.
- This product contains phenylalanine and should not be used by those with phenylketonuria.
- Consult your pharmacist or physician for further information.

CAL SUP 600 PLUS
(calcium supplement with multivitamins)

Manufacturer: 3M Company
Dosage Form: Tablets
Ingredients:

elemental calcium	600 mg
vitamin D	200 IU
vitamin C	30 mg

Comments: This product contains no sugar, salt, or lactose.

Supplement Product Profiles

CALTRATE 600 (calcium supplement)

Manufacturer: Lederle Laboratories
Dosage Form: Tablets
Ingredients:

elemental calcium	600 mg

Comments: No sugar, salt, or lactose is contained in this supplement.

CENTRUM (multivitamin/mineral supplement)

Manufacturer: Lederle Laboratories
Dosage form: Tablets
Ingredients:

vitamin A	5,000 IU
vitamin E	30 IU
vitamin C	90 mg
folic acid	400 µg
thiamin (B_1)	2.25 mg
riboflavin (B_2)	2.6 mg
niacinamide	20 mg
vitamin B_6	3 mg
vitamin B_{12}	9 µg
vitamin D	400 IU
biotin	45 µg
pantothenic acid	10 mg
calcium	162 mg
phosphorus	125 mg
iodine	150 µg
iron	100 mg
magnesium	100 mg
copper	2 mg
manganese	5 mg

potassium	30 mg
chloride	27.2 mg
chromium	25 µg
molybdenum	25 µg
selenium	25 µg
zinc	15 mg
vitamin K$_1$	25 µg

Comments:

- Accidental iron poisoning is a real possibility, especially with young children. *Be sure all nutrient supplements are stored out of their reach.*

- This product contains greater than 100 percent of the U.S. RDA for vitamin C, thiamin, riboflavin, B$_6$, B$_{12}$, and iron.

COD LIVER OIL CONCENTRATE
(multivitamin supplement)

Manufacturer: Schering Corporation
Dosage Forms: Capsules, chewable tablets
Ingredients:

Capsules:

vitamin A	10,000 IU
vitamin D	200 IU

Tablets:

vitamin A	4,000 IU
vitamin D	200 IU

Comments:

- Capsules contain greater than 100 percent of the U.S. RDA for vitamin A.

- Tablets contain FD&C Yellow No. 5 (tartrazine) as a color additive. Persons sensitive to tartrazine or aspirin should consult their physician before using this supplement.

DAYALETS (multivitamin supplement)

Manufacturer: Abbott Laboratories
Dosage form: Tablets
Ingredients:

vitamin A	5,000 IU
vitamin D	400 IU
vitamin E	30 IU
vitamin C	60 mg
folic acid	0.4 mg
thiamin (B_1)	1.5 mg
riboflavin (B_2)	1.7 mg
niacin	20 mg
vitamin B_6	2 mg
vitamin B_{12}	6 μg

Comments: This supplement contains no sugar.

DAYALETS PLUS IRON
(multivitamin supplement plus iron)

Manufacturer: Abbott Laboratories
Dosage form: Tablets
Ingredients: DAYALETS PLUS IRON contains the same ingredients as DAYALETS, plus 18 mg of iron.
Comments:

- No sugar is contained in this product.
- Accidental iron poisoning is a real possibility, especially with young children. *Be sure all nutrient supplements are stored out of their reach.*

EFAMOL PMS
(multivitamin/mineral supplement)

Manufacturer: Murdock Pharmaceuticals, Inc.
Dosage form: Capsules
Ingredients:

vitamin B_6	21 mg
vitamin E	12 IU
vitamin C	100 mg
calcium	20 mg
magnesium	30 mg
zinc	3 mg

Comments:
- This product contains no sugar, sodium, starch, artificial colors, flavors or preservatives.
- The manufacturer recommends doses up to six capsules a day. One capsule contains a megadose of B_6 (ten or more times the U.S. RDA) and over 100 percent of the U.S. RDA for vitamin C. Daily multiple doses could pose the risk of overdose.

ENER-B (vitamin B_{12} supplement)

Manufacturer: Nature's Bounty, Inc.
Dosage form: Intra-nasal gel
Ingredients:

vitamin B_{12}	400 µg

Comments:
- Each nasal applicator delivers $1/10$ cc of gel into the nose which adheres to the mucous membranes.
- Each application contains a megadose of vitamin B_{12} (ten or more times the U.S. RDA).

Supplement Product Profiles

FEMIRON (iron supplement)

Manufacturer: Beecham Products
Dosage form: Tablets
Ingredients:

Iron	20 mg

Comments:

- Accidental iron poisoning is a real possibility, especially with young children. *Be sure to keep all supplements stored out of their reach.*
- Iron interacts with antacids and oral tetracycline antibiotics, reducing absorption of the drugs.
- A darkened stool may result from use of this supplement.
- This product should not be used by alcoholics or by individuals with chronic liver or pancreatic disease.
- This supplement contains more than 100 percent of the U.S. RDA for iron.
- Consult your pharmacist or physician for more information.

FEMIRON PLUS
(iron supplement plus multivitamins)

Manufacturer: Beecham Products
Dosage form: Tablets
Ingredients:

iron	20 mg
vitamin A	5,000 IU
vitamin D	400 IU

thiamin (B_1)	1.5 mg
riboflavin (B_2)	1.7 mg
niacin	20 mg
vitamin C	60 mg
vitamin B_6	2 mg
vitamin B_{12}	6 µg
pantothenic acid	10 mg
folic acid	0.4 mg
vitamin E	15 IU

Comments:

- Accidental iron poisoning is a real possibility, especially with young children. *Be sure to keep all supplements stored out of their reach.*

- A darkened stool may result from use of this supplement.

- This product should not be used by alcoholics or individuals with chronic liver or pancreatic disease.

- This supplement contains more than 100 percent of the U.S. RDA for iron.

- Iron interacts with antacids and oral tetracycline antibiotics, reducing absorption of these drugs.

- Consult your pharmacist or physician for more information.

FEOSOL (iron supplement)

Manufacturer: SmithKline Consumer Products
Dosage form: Capsules, tablets
Ingredients:

| Capsules: | elemental iron | 50 mg |
| Tablets: | elemental iron | 65 mg |

Supplement Product Profiles

Comments:

- Accidental iron poisoning is a real possibility, especially with young children. *Be sure to keep all supplements stored out of their reach.*
- This product may cause gastrointestinal discomfort and nausea. These side effects may be minimized by taking the supplement with meals.
- Other side effects include constipation or diarrhea.
- The supplement contains more than 100 percent of the U.S. RDA for iron.
- Capsules contain FD&C Red No. 40, a food coloring whose safety is in question.

FEOSOL ELIXIR (iron supplement)

Manufacturer: SmithKline Consumer Products
Dosage form: Liquid
Ingredients:

    elemental iron   44 mg

Comments:

- This product contains 5 percent alcohol.
- Accidental iron poisoning is a real possibility, especially with young children. *Be sure to keep all supplements stored out of their reach.*
- This product may cause gastrointestinal discomfort and nausea. These side effects may be minimized by taking the supplement with meals.
- Other side effects include constipation or diarrhea and temporary staining of the teeth.
- This supplement contains more than 100 percent of the U.S. RDA for iron.
- Iron interacts with oral tetracycline antibiotics, reducing absorption of the drug.

- Consult your pharmacist or physician for more information.

FERANCEE (iron supplement with vitamin C)

Manufacturer: Stuart Pharmaceuticals
Dosage form: Chewable tablets
Ingredients:

iron	67 mg
vitamin C	150 mg

Comments:
- Accidental iron poisoning is a real possibility, especially with young children. *Be sure to keep all supplements stored out of their reach.*
- A darkened stool may result from use of this supplement.
- This product contains more than 100 percent of the U.S. RDA for iron and vitamin C.

FERANCEE-HP
(iron supplement with vitamin C)

Manufacturer: Stuart Pharmaceuticals
Dosage form: Tablets
Ingredients:

iron	110 mg
vitamin C	600 mg

Comments:
- Accidental iron poisoning is a real possibility, especially with young children. *Be sure to keep all supplements stored out of their reach.*

Supplement Product Profiles

- This is a high-potency formulation, not recommended for children under 12 years of age.
- This product may cause a darkened stool and an upset stomach.
- This supplement contains more than 100 percent of the U.S. RDA for iron and vitamin C.
- It also contains FD&C Red No. 40, a food coloring whose safety is in question.

FER-IN-SOL (iron supplement)

Manufacturer: Mead Johnson Nutritional Division
Dosage form: Drops, liquid, capsules
Ingredients:

Drops:	elemental iron	15 mg
Liquid:	elemental iron	18 mg
Capsules:	elemental iron	60 mg

Comments:
- The drops contain 0.02 percent alcohol.
- The liquid contains 5 percent alcohol.
- Both the drops and liquid are used as a pediatric iron supplement.
- Capsules are used as an adult supplement often recommended for women who are pregnant or breast-feeding.
- Accidental iron poisoning is a real possibility, especially with young children. *Be sure to keep all supplements stored out of their reach.*
- This product is recommended for use immediately after meals.
- Side effects include darkened stool and temporary gum discoloration.

- Capsules contain more than 100 percent of the U.S. RDA for iron.

FERGON (iron supplement)

Manufacturer: Winthrop-Breon Laboratories
Dosage form: Capsules, tablets, liquid
Ingredients:

Capsules:	elemental iron	50 mg
Tablets:	ferrous iron	36 mg
Liquid:	ferrous iron	34 mg

Comments:

- The liquid form contains saccharin and 7 percent alcohol.
- Accidental iron poisoning is a real possibility, especially with young children. *Be sure to keep all supplements stored our of their reach.*
- Occasionally, this product may cause nausea, abdominal cramps, constipation, or diarrhea.
- Iron interacts with oral tetracycline antibiotics, reducing their absorption.
- Consult your pharmacist or physician for further information.
- This product provides greater than 100 percent of the U.S. RDA for iron.

FLINTSTONES WITH EXTRA C (multivitamin supplement)

Manufacturer: Miles Laboratories, Inc.
Dosage form: Chewable tablets

Supplement Product Profiles

Ingredients:

vitamin A	2,500 IU
vitamin D	400 IU
vitamin E	15 IU
vitamin C	250 mg
folic acid	0.3 mg
thiamin (B_1)	1.05 mg
riboflavin (B_2)	1.20 mg
niacin	13.50 mg
vitamin B_6	1.05 mg
vitamin B_{12}	4.5 μg

Comments:

● For children 2 to 4 years of age, this product contains greater than 100 percent of the U.S. RDA for vitamin E, vitamin C, folic acid, thiamin, riboflavin, niacin, B_6, and B_{12}.

● For children over 4 years of age, this product contains greater than 100 percent of the U.S. RDA for vitamin C.

● Long-term use of chewable vitamin C tablets has been linked to dental erosion.

● This product contains phenylalanine and should not be used by children who have phenylketonuria.

FLINTSTONES WITH IRON
(multivitamin supplement with iron)

Manufacturer: Miles Laboratories, Inc.
Dosage form: Chewable tablets

Ingredients:

vitamin A	2,500 IU
vitamin D	400 IU
vitamin E	15 IU
vitamin C	60 mg
folic acid	0.3 mg
thiamine (B_1)	1.05 mg
riboflavin (B_2)	1.20 mg
niacin	13.50 mg
vitamin B_6	1.05 mg
vitamin B_{12}	4.5 µg
iron	15 mg

Comments:

- Accidental iron poisoning is a real possibility especially with young children. *Be sure to keep all supplements stored out of their reach.*

- For children 2 to 4 years of age, this product contains more that 100 percent of the U.S. RDA for vitamin E, vitamin C, folic acid, thiamin, riboflavin, niacin, B_6, B_{12}, and iron.

- This product contains phenylalanine and should not be used by children who have phenylketonuria.

GERIPLEX-FS KAPSEALS
(multivitamin/mineral supplement and stool softener)

Manufacturer: Parke-Davis
Dosage form: Capsules
Ingredients:

vitamin A	5,000 IU
vitamin C	50 mg

Supplement Product Profiles

thiamin (B_1)	5 mg
riboflavin (B_2)	5 mg
vitamin B_{12})	2 µg
choline	20 mg
niacin	15 mg
vitamin E	5 IU
iron	6 mg
copper	4 mg
manganese	4 mg
zinc	2 mg
calcium	200 mg

Comments:
- This product contains the stool softener docusate sodium.
- Consult your physician before routinely taking a supplement with a laxative effect.
- This supplement contains more than 100 percent of the U.S. RDA for thiamin, riboflavin, and copper.
- Contains FD&C Red No. 3, whose safety as a food colorant is in question.

GERIPLEX-FS
(multivitamin plus iron with a stool softener)

Manufacturer: Parke-Davis
Dosage form: Liquid
Ingredients:

thiamin (B_1)	1.2 mg
riboflavin (B_2)	1.7 mg
vitamin B_6	1 mg
vitamin B_{12}	5 µg

niacin	15 mg
iron	15 mg

Comments:
- This product contains a stool softener.
- Consult your physician before routinely taking a supplement with a laxative effect.
- This product contains glucose, sugar, sorbitol, saccharin, and 18 percent alcohol.
- It also contains FD&C Red No. 40, whose safety as a food colorant is in question.
- Accidental iron poisoning is a real possibility, especially with young children. *Keep all supplements stored out of their reach.*

GERITOL (iron and multivitamin tonic)

Manufacturer: Beecham Products
Dosage form: Liquid
Ingredients:

iron	50 mg
thiamin (B_1)	2.5 mg
riboflavin (B_2)	2.5 mg
niacin	50 mg
pantothenic acid	2 mg
vitamin B_6	0.5 mg
vitamin B_{12}	0.75 μg
choline	50 mg

Comments:
- This product contains more than 100 percent of the U.S. RDA for iron, thiamin, riboflavin, and niacin.

Supplement Product Profiles

- It contains alcohol, which may accelerate the absorption of iron.
- This supplement should not be used by alcoholics or individuals with chronic liver or pancreatic disease.
- Accidental iron poisoning is a real possibility, especially with young children. *Keep all supplements stored out of their reach.*
- This product may cause darkening of the stool.

GERITOL COMPLETE
(multivitamin/mineral supplement)

Manufacturer: Beecham Products
Dosage form: Tablets
Ingredients:

vitamin A	5,000 IU
vitamin E	30 IU
vitamin C	60 mg
folic acid	400 µg
thiamin (B_1)	1.5 mg
riboflavin (B_2)	1.7 mg
niacin	20 mg
vitamin B_6	2 mg
vitamin B_{12}	6 µg
vitamin D	400 IU
biotin	300 µg
pantothenic acid	10 mg
vitamin K	50 µg
calcium	162 mg
phosphorus	125 mg
iodine	150 µg
iron	30 mg

magnesium	100 mg.
copper	2 mg
manganese	7.5 mg
potassium	37.5 mg
chloride	34.1 mg
chromium	15 µg
molybdenum	15 µg
selenium	15 µg
zinc	15 mg
nickel	5 µg
silicon	10 µg

Comments:

- This product contains more than 100 percent of the U.S. RDA for iron.
- Accidental iron poisoning is a real possibility, especially with young children. *Keep all supplements stored out of their reach.*
- This supplement should not be used by alcoholics or individuals with chronic liver or pancreatic disease.
- This product contains FD&C Red No. 40, whose safety as a food colorant is in question.

GEVRABON
(multivitamin/mineral supplement)

Manufacturer: Lederle Laboratories
Dosage form: Liquid
Ingredients:

thiamin (B₁)	5 mg
riboflavin (B₂)	2.5 mg
niacin	50 mg
vitamin B₆	1 mg

Supplement Product Profiles

vitamin B_{12}	1 μg
pantothenic acid	10 mg
iodine	100 μg
iron	15 mg
magnesium	2 mg
zinc	2 mg
choline	100 mg
manganese	2 mg

Comments:

- This product provides more than 100 percent of the U.S. RDA for thiamin, riboflavin, niacin, and pantothenic acid.
- Accidental iron poisoning is a real possibility, especially with young children. *Keep all supplements stored out of their reach.*
- This supplement contains 18 percent alcohol.

GEVRAL (multivitamin/mineral supplement)

Manufacturer: Lederle Laboratories
Dosage form: Tablets
Ingredients:

vitamin A	5,000 IU
vitamin E	30 IU
vitamin C	60 mg
folic acid	400 μg
thiamin (B_1)	1.5 mg
riboflavin (B_2)	1.7 mg
niacin	20 mg
vitamin B_6	2 mg
vitamin B_{12}	6 μg

calcium	162 mg
phosphorus	125 mg
iodine	150 μg
iron	18 mg
magnesium	100 mg

Comments: Accidental iron poisoning is a real possibility, especially with young children. *Keep all supplements out of their reach.*

GEVRAL T
(multivitamin/mineral supplement)

Manufacturer: Lederle Laboratories
Dosage form: Tablets
Ingredients:

vitamin A	5,000 IU
vitamin E	45 IU
vitamin C	90 mg
folic acid	400 μg
thiamin (B_1)	2.25 mg
riboflavin	2.6 mg
niacin	30 mg
vitamin B_6	3 mg
vitamin B_{12}	9 μg
vitamin D	400 IU
calcium	162 mg
phosphorus	125 mg
iodine	225 μg
iron	27 mg
magnesium	100 mg
copper	1.5 mg
zinc	22.5 mg

Supplement Product Profiles

Comments:

- This product provides greater than 100 percent of the U.S. RDA for vitamin E, vitamin C, thiamin, riboflavin, niacin, B_6, B_{12}, iodine, iron, and zinc.
- Accidental iron poisoning is a real possibility, especially with young children. *Keep all supplements stored out of their reach.*

INCREMIN (multivitamin plus iron)

Manufacturer: Lederle Laboratories
Dosage form: Liquid
Ingredients:

elemental iron	30 mg
thiamin (B_1)	10 mg
vitamin B_6	5 mg
vitamin B_{12}	25 µg

Comments:

- This product provides more than 100 percent of the U.S. RDA for iron, thiamin, B_6, and B_{12}.
- Accidental iron poisoning is a real possibility, especially with young children. *Keep all supplements out of their reach.*
- This supplement contains 0.75 percent alcohol.
- It also contains sorbitol.

KLB$_6$ GRAPEFRUIT DIET
(diet aide plus B$_6$)

Manufacturer: Nature's Bounty, Inc.
Dosage form: Tablets

Ingredients:

vitamin B$_6$	5 mg

Comments:

- This product contains grapefruit extract, gluconmannan, lecithin, kelp, cider vinegar, uva ursi and phenylalanine (an amino acid), fortified with vitamin B$_6$.

- To date, there's no research to prove that this combination is effective for weight loss. Uva ursi is an herb that functions as a diuretic (water pill), which may lead to temporary water weight loss.

- This product provides over 100 percent of the U.S. RDA for B$_6$ in one tablet. The recommended dosage suggests four tablets a day, which would provide a megadose of B$_6$ (ten or more times the U.S. RDA).

MARLYN PMS
(multivitamin/mineral supplement)

Manufacturer: Marlyn Co., Inc.
Dosage form: Tablets, capsules
Ingredients:

vitamin A	5,000 IU
vitamin D	400 IU
vitamin E	200 IU
thiamin (B$_1$)	25 mg
riboflavin (B$_2$)	25 mg
niacin	25 mg
vitamin B$_6$	125 mg
vitamin B$_{12}$	50 μg
biotin	25 μg
pantothenic acid	25 mg

Supplement Product Profiles

folic acid	200 μg
choline	50 mg
inositol	50 mg
para-aminobenzoic acid	50 mg
vitamin C	500 mg
lemon bioflavonoids	100 mg
hesperidin	100 mg
iron	9 mg
calcium	200 mg
phosphorus	155 mg
iodine	75 μg
zinc	7.5 mg
copper	1 mg
manganese	5 mg
potassium	25 mg
chromium	1 μg
selenium	50 μg
magnesium	250 mg

Comments:

- This product provides over 100 percent of the U.S. RDA of vitamin E, B_{12}, pantothenic acid, and vitamin C. Thiamin, riboflavin, and B_6 are provided in ranges that would be considered megadoses (ten or more times the U.S. RDA).
- This supplement contains no sugar and starch.
- Accidental iron poisoning is a real possibility, especially with young children. *Keep all supplements stored out of their reach.*

MEGA-B (multivitamin B supplement)

Manufacturer: Arco Pharmaceuticals
Dosage form: Tablets

Ingredients:

thiamin (B_1)	100 mg
riboflavin (B_2)	100 mg
vitamin B_6	100 mg
vitamin B_{12}	100 µg
choline	100 mg
inositol	100 mg
niacin	100 mg
folic acid	100 µg
pantothenic acid	100 mg
biotin	100 µg
para-aminobenzoic acid	100 mg

Comments:

- This product provides over 100 percent of the U.S. RDA for niacin.
- Thiamin, riboflavin, B_6, B_{12}, pantothenic acid, and biotin are provided in ranges that would be considered megadoses (ten or more times the U.S. RDA).

MOL-IRON (iron supplement plus vitamin C)

Manufacturer: Schering Corporation
Dosage form: Tablets
Ingredients:

elemental iron	39 mg
vitamin C	75 mg

Comments:

- This product provides more than 100 percent of the U.S. RDA for iron and vitamin C.
- Accidental iron poisoning is a real possibility, especially with young children. *Keep all supplements stored out of their reach.*

Supplement Product Profiles

• This supplement contains FD&C Red No. 40, whose safety as a food colorant is in question.

MYADEC (multivitamin/mineral supplement)

Manufacturer: Parke-Davis
Dosage form: Tablets
Ingredients:

vitamin A	9,000 IU
vitamin D	400 IU
vitamin E	30 IU
vitamin C	90 mg
folic acid	400 μg
thiamin (B_1)	10 mg
riboflavin (B_2)	10 mg
niacin	20 mg
vitamin B_6	5 mg
vitamin B_{12}	10 μg
pantothenic acid	20 mg
vitamin K	25 μg
biotin	45 μg
iodine	150 μg
iron	30 mg
magnesium	100 mg
copper	3 mg
zinc	15 mg
manganese	7.5 mg
calcium	70 mg
phosphorus	54 mg
potassium	8 mg
selenium	15 μg
molybdenum	10 μg
chromium	15 μg

Comments:

- This product provides more than 100 percent of the U.S. RDA for vitamin A, vitamin C, thiamin, riboflavin, B_6, B_{12}, pantothenic acid, iron, and copper.
- Accidental iron poisoning is a real possibility, especially with young children. *Keep all supplements stored out of their reach.*

NATABEC KAPSEALS
(multivitamin/mineral supplement)

Manufacturer: Parke-Davis
Dosage form: Capsules
Ingredients:

vitamin A	4,000 IU
vitamin D	400 IU
vitamin C	50 mg
thiamin (B_1)	3 mg
riboflavin (B_2)	2 mg
niacin	10 mg
vitamin B_6	3 mg
vitamin B_{12}	5 μg
calcium	600 mg
iron	30 mg

Comments:

- This product provides greater than 100 percent of the U.S. RDA for thiamin, riboflavin, B_6, and iron.
- Accidental iron poisoning is a real possibility, especially with small children. *Keep all supplements stored out of their reach.*

Supplement Product Profiles

NATURE MADE VITAMIN C
(vitamin supplement)

Manufacturer: Nature Made Nutritional Products
Dosage form: Tablets
Ingredients:
  vitamin C available in 250 mg, 500 mg, and
  1,000 mg tablets.
Comments:
- 250 and 500 mg tablets provide greater than 100 percent of the U.S. RDA.
- 1,000 mg tablets would be considered a mega-dose (ten or more times the U.S. RDA).

NATURE MADE VITAMIN E
(vitamin supplement)

Manufacturer: Nature Made Nutritional Products
Dosage form: Capsules
Ingredients:
  vitamin E available in 200 IU, 400 IU, and
  1,000 IU capsules.
Comments:
- 200 IU and 400 IU capsules provide greater than 100 percent of the U.S. RDA.
- 1,000 IU capsules would be considered a mega-dose (ten or more times the U.S. RDA).

NICOTINEX ELIXIR (niacin supplement)

Manufacturer: Fleming & Company
Dosage form: Liquid
Ingredients:

niacin   50 mg

Comments:

- This product provides greater than 100 percent of the U.S. RDA for niacin.
- It may cause flushing of the skin.
- This supplement contains 14 percent alcohol.
- It should not be used by individuals who have gout or ulcers.

ONE-A-DAY ESSENTIAL VITAMINS (multivitamin supplement)

Manufacturer: Miles Laboratories, Inc.
Dosage form: Tablets
Ingredients:

vitamin A	5,000 IU
vitamin C	60 mg
thiamin (B_1)	1.5 mg
riboflavin (B_2)	1.7 mg
niacin	20 mg
vitamin D	400 IU
vitamin E	30 IU
vitamin B_6	2 mg
folic acid	400 µg
vitamin B_{12}	6 µg
pantothenic acid	10 mg

Supplement Product Profiles

Comments: All vitamins in this supplement are supplied in amounts that equal 100 percent of the U.S. RDA.

ONE-A-DAY MAXIMUM FORMULA
(multivitamin/mineral supplement)

Manufacturer: Miles Laboratories, Inc.
Dosage form: Tablets
Ingredients:

vitamin A	5,000 IU
vitamin C	60 mg
thiamin (B_1)	1.5 mg
riboflavin (B_2)	1.7 mg
niacin	20 mg
vitamin D	400 IU
vitamin E	30 IU
vitamin B_6	2 mg
folic acid	0.4 mg
vitamin B_{12}	6 µg
biotin	30 µg
pantothenic acid	10 mg
vitamin K	50 µg
elemental iron	18 mg
calcium	129.6 mg
phosphorus	100 mg
iodine	150 µg

Comments:
- This product provides 100 percent of the U.S. RDA for all nutrients except biotin, calcium, and phosphorus, which are provided in lesser amounts.
- Accidental iron poisoning is a real possibility, espe-

cially with young children. *Store all supplements out of their reach.*

ONE-A-DAY PLUS EXTRA C
(multivitamin supplement)

Manufacturer: Miles Laboratories
Dosage form: Tablets
Ingredients:

vitamin A	5,000 IU
vitamin C	300 mg
thiamin (B_1)	1.5 mg
riboflavin (B_2)	1.7 mg
niacin	20 mg
vitamin D	400 IU
vitamin E	30 IU
vitamin B_6	2 mg
folic acid	400 μg
vitamin B_{12}	6 μg
pantothenic acid	10 mg

Comments: This product provides 100 percent of the U.S. RDA for all nutrients except vitamin C, which is provided in excess of 100 percent of the recommended dietary allowance.

OPTILETS 500 (multivitamin supplement)

Manufacturer: Abbott Laboratories
Dosage form: Tablets
Ingredients:

vitamin C	500 mg
niacin	100 mg

pantothenic acid	20 mg
thiamin (B_1)	15 mg
riboflavin (B_2)	10 mg
vitamin B_6	5 mg
vitamin A	10,000 IU
vitamin B_{12}	12 μg
vitamin D	400 IU
vitamin E	30 IU

Comments:

- This product provides greater than 100 percent of the U.S. RDA for vitamin C, niacin, pantothenic acid, riboflavin, B_6, vitamin A, and B_{12}.
- Thiamin is provided in a megadose amount (ten or more times the U.S. RDA).

OPTILETS-M-500
(multivitamin/mineral supplement)

Manufacturer: Abbott Laboratories
Dosage form: Tablets
Ingredients:

vitamin C	500 mg
niacin	100 mg
pantothenic acid	20 mg
thiamin (B_1)	15 mg
riboflavin (B_2)	10 mg
vitamin B_6	5 mg
vitamin A	10,000 IU
vitamin B_{12}	12 μg
vitamin D	400 IU

vitamin E	30 IU
magnesium	80 mg
iron	20 mg
copper	2 mg
zinc	1.5 mg
manganese	1 mg
iodine	150 μg

Comments:

- This product provides greater than 100 percent of the U.S. RDA for vitamin C, niacin, pantothenic acid, riboflavin, B_6, vitamin A, B_{12}, and iron.
- Thiamin is provided in a megadose amount (ten or more times the U.S. RDA).
- Accidental iron poisoning is a real possibility, especially with young children. *Keep all supplements stored out of their reach.*

OREXIN SOFTTAB
(B-complex multivitamin supplement)

Manufacturer: Stuart Pharmaceuticals
Dosage form: Tablets
Ingredients:

thiamin (B_1)	10 mg
vitamin B_6	5 mg
vitamin B_{12}	25 μg

Comments:

- This product provides greater than 100 percent of the U.S. RDA for each nutrient.
- It contains mannitol and saccharin.

Supplement Product Profiles

OS-CAL 500 CHEWABLE TABLETS
(calcium supplement)

Manufacturer: Marion Laboratories, Inc.
Dosage form: Chewable tablets
Ingredients:
    elemental calcium   500 mg
Comments: The calcium source is calcium carbonate.

OS-CAL 500 TABLETS (calcium supplement)

Manufacturer: Marion Laboratories, Inc.
Dosage form: Tablets
Ingredients:
    elemental calcium   500 mg
Comments: The calcium source is crushed oyster shell powder.

OS-CAL 250+D TABLETS
(calcium supplement with vitamin D)

Manufacturer: Marion Laboratories, Inc.
Dosage form: Tablets
Ingredients:
    elemental calcium   250 mg
    vitamin D   125 IU
Comments: The calcium source is crushed oyster shell powder.

OS-CAL 500 + D TABLETS
(calcium supplement with vitamin D)

Manufacturer: Marion Laboratories, Inc.
Dosage form: Tablets
Ingredients:

elemental calcium	500 mg
vitamin D	125 IU

Comments: The calcium source is crushed oyster shell powder.

OS-CAL FORTE TABLETS
(multivitamin/mineral supplement)

Manufacturer: Marion Laboratories, Inc.
Dosage form: Tablets
Ingredients:

vitamin A	1,668 IU
vitamin D	125 IU
thiamin (B_1)	1.7 mg
riboflavin	1.7 mg
vitamin B_6	2 mg
vitamin B_{12}	1.6 µg
vitamin C	50 mg
vitamin E	0.8 IU
niacin	15 mg
calcium	250 mg
iron	5 mg
magnesium	1.6 mg

| manganese | 0.3 mg |
| zinc | 0.5 mg |

Comments:

- The calcium source is crushed oyster shell powder.
- This product contains slightly more than 100 percent of the U.S. RDA for thiamin.
- Accidental iron poisoning is a real possibility, especially with young children. *Keep all supplements stored out of their reach.*

OS-CAL PLUS TABLETS
(multivitamin/mineral supplement)

Manufacturer: Marion Laboratories, Inc.
Dosage form: Tablets
Ingredients:

elemental calcium	250 mg
vitamin D	125 IU
vitamin A	1,666 IU
vitamin C	33 mg
riboflavin (B$_2$)	0.66 mg
thiamin (B$_1$)	0.5 mg
vitamin B$_6$	0.5 mg
niacin	3.33 mg
iron	16.6 mg
zinc	0.75 mg
manganese	0.75 mg

Comments:

- The calcium source is crushed oyster shell powder.
- Accidental iron poisoning is a real possibility, especially with young children. *Keep all supplements stored out of their reach.*

Supplement Product Profiles

POLY-VI-SOL (multivitamin supplement)

Manufacturer: Mead Johnson Nutritional Division
Dosage form: Liquid, chewable tablets
Ingredients:

Liquid:

vitamin A	1,500 IU
vitamin D	400 IU
vitamin E	5 IU
vitamin C	35 mg
thiamin (B_1)	0.5 mg
riboflavin (B_2)	0.6 mg
niacin	8 mg
vitamin B_6	0.4 mg
vitamin B_{12}	2 µg

Chewable tablets:

vitamin A	2,500 IU
vitamin D	400 IU
vitamin E	15 IU
vitamin C	60 mg
folic acid	300 µg
thiamin (B_1)	1.05 mg
riboflavin (B_2)	1.2 mg
niacin	13.5 mg
vitamin B_6	1.05 mg
vitamin B_{12}	4.5 µg

Comments:

- The liquid supplement provides 100 percent of the U.S. RDA for infants, with lesser amounts provided if used for an older child or adult.
- The chewable tablets provide greater that 100 percent of the U.S. RDA for vitamin E, vitamin C, folic acid, thiamin, riboflavin, niacin, B_6, and B_{12} for children under age four. For children over age

Supplement Product Profiles

4, 100 percent or less of the U.S. RDA is provided for each nutrient.

POLY-VI-SOL WITH IRON
(multivitamin supplement with iron)

Manufacturer: Mead Johnson Nutritional Division
Dosage form: Liquid
Ingredients:

vitamin A	1,500 IU
vitamin D	400 IU
vitamin E	5 IU
thiamin (B_1)	0.5 mg
riboflavin (B_2)	0.6 mg
niacin	8 mg
vitamin B_6	0.4 mg
iron	10 mg

Comments:

- This product provides 100 percent of the U.S. RDA for infants for each vitamin and a lesser amount for iron.
- Accidental iron poisoning is a real possibility, especially with young children. *Keep all supplements stored out of their reach.*
- This supplement may cause darkened stools or temporary discoloration of the gums.

POLY-VI-SOL WITH MINERALS
(multivitamin/mineral supplement)

Manufacturer: Mead Johnson Nutritional Division
Dosage form: Chewable tablets

Ingredients:
Each tablet provides the same amount of vitamins as Poly-Vi-Sol chewable vitamins along with:

iron	12 mg
zinc	8 mg
copper	0.8 mg

Comments:

- This product provides greater than 100 percent of the U.S. RDA for vitamin E, folic acid, thiamin, riboflavin, niacin, B_6, B_{12}, and iron for children under age 4. For children over the age of 4, 100 percent of the U.S. RDA or less is provided for each nutrient.

- Accidental iron poisoning is a real possibility, especially for young children. *Keep all supplements stored out of their reach.*

POSTURE (calcium supplement)

Manufacturer: Ayerst Laboratories
Dosage form: Tablets, 300 mg and 600 mg
Ingredients:
300 mg tablet provides:

elemental calcium	300 mg

600 mg tablet provides:

elemental calcium	600 mg

Comments: The calcium source is tricalcium phosphate.

Supplement Product Profiles

POSTURE-D
(calcium supplement plus vitamin D)

Manufacturer: Ayerst Laboratories
Dosage form: Tablets, 300 mg and 600 mg tablets
Ingredients:
    300 mg tablet provides:

elemental calcium	300 mg
vitamin D	125 IU

    600 mg tablet provides:

elemental calcium	600 mg
vitamin D	125 IU

Comments: The calcium source is tricalcium phosphate.

PROBEC-T (vitamin B complex
supplement plus vitamin C)

Manufacturer: Stuart Pharmaceuticals
Dosage form: Tablets
Ingredients:

vitamin C	600 mg
thiamin (B_1)	15 mg
riboflavin (B_2)	10 mg
vitamin B_6	5 mg
vitamin B_{12}	5 µg
niacin	100 mg
pantothenic acid	20 mg

Comments:
- This product provides greater than 100 percent of the U.S. RDA for vitamin C, riboflavin, B_6, niacin, and pantothenic acid.

- This supplement provides a megadose for thiamin (ten or more times the U.S. RDA).

SCOTT'S EMULSION
(vitamin A and D supplement)

Manufacturer: Beecham Products
Dosage form: Liquid
Ingredients:

vitamin A	5,000 IU
vitamin D	400 IU

Comments: The nutrient source is cod liver oil.

SHAKLEE CALCIUM COMPLEX
(multimineral supplement)

Manufacturer: Shaklee Corporation
Dosage form: Tablets
Ingredients:

calcium	400 mg
magnesium	13.3 mg
copper	0.66 mg
zinc	0.5 mg
manganese	0.5 mg

Comments: The calcium sources are limestone, calcium lactate, and calcium gluconate.

Supplement Product Profiles

SHAKLEE CHEWABLE CALCIUM COMPLEX
(multimineral supplement)

Manufacturer: Shaklee Corporation
Dosage form: Chewable tablets
Ingredients:

calcium	333 mg
magnesium	13.3 mg
copper	0.66 mg
zinc	0.5 mg
manganese	0.5 mg

Comments:
- The calcium sources are calcium carbonate, calcium lactate, and calcium gluconate.
- This product contains nonfat dry milk solids.

SIGTAB (multivitamin supplement)

Manufacturer: The Upjohn Company
Dosage form: Tablets
Ingredients:

vitamin A	5,000 IU
vitamin D	400 IU
vitamin E	15 IU
vitamin C	333 mg
folic acid	400 μg
thiamin (B_1)	10.3 mg
riboflavin (B_2)	10 mg
niacin	100 mg

vitamin B_6	6 mg
vitamin B_{12}	18 µg
pantothenic acid	20 mg

Comments:

- This product provides greater than 100 percent of the U.S. RDA for vitamin C, thiamin, riboflavin, niacin, B_6, B_{12}, and pantothenic acid.
- This supplement contains sucrose.

SIMRON (iron supplement)

Manufacturer: Merrell Dow Pharmaceuticals, Inc.
Dosage form: Capsules
Ingredients:

| elemental iron | 10 mg |

Comments:

- Accidental iron poisoning is a real possibility, especially with young children. *Keep all supplements stored out of their reach.*
- This product contains FD&C Red No. 3 and Red No. 40. The safety of both of these food colorants is in question.
- This supplement should not be used by those who have hemochromatosis (a condition associated with increased iron storage).
- Iron interferes with the absorption of tetracycline antibiotics and may reduce the effectiveness of the drug.
- Consult your pharmacist or physician for further information.

SIMRON PLUS
(iron plus multivitamin supplement)

Manufacturer: Merrell Dow Pharmaceuticals, Inc.
Dosage form: Capsules
Ingredients:

elemental iron	10 mg
vitamin C	50 mg
vitamin B_{12}	3.33 μg
vitamin B_6	1.0 mg
folic acid	100 μg

Comments:

- Accidental iron poisoning is a real possibility, especially with young children. *Keep all supplements stored out of their reach.*

- This product contains FD&C Red No. 40 and Red No. 3. The safety of both of these food colorants is in question.

- This supplement should not be used by those who have hemochromatosis (a condition associated with increased iron storage).

- Iron interferes with the absorption of tetracycline antibiotics and may reduce the effectiveness of the drug.

- Consult your pharmacist or physician for further information.

SMURF (multivitamin supplement)

Manufacturer: Mead Johnson Nutritional Division
Dosage form: Chewable tablets

Ingredients:

vitamin A	2,500 IU
vitamin D	400 IU
vitamin E	15 IU
vitamin C	60 mg
folic acid	300 µg
thiamin (B_1)	1.05 mg
riboflavin (B_2)	1.2 mg
niacin	13.5 mg
vitamin B_6	1.05 mg
vitamin B_{12}	4.5 µg

Comments:

- This product provides greater than 100 percent of the U.S. RDA for vitamin C, folic acid, thiamin, riboflavin, niacin, B_6, and B_{12} for children under 4 years of age.
- This product provides 100 percent or less of the U.S. RDA for each nutrient for children age 4 or older.

SMURF WITH IRON AND ZINC
(multivitamin/mineral supplement)

Manufacturer: Mead Johnson Nutritional Division
Dosage form: Chewable tablets
Ingredients:

Contains the same nutrient amounts as SMURF, with the addition of 12 mg of iron and 8 mg of zinc.

Comments:

- Same as for SMURF.
- Accidental iron poisoning is a real possibility, especially with young children. *Keep all supplements out of their reach.*

Supplement Product Profiles

SOFT STRESS
(multivitamin/mineral supplement)

Manufacturer: Marlyn Co., Inc.
Dosage form: Capsules
Ingredients:

vitamin A as beta-carotene,	15 mg
which is equivalent to	25,000 IU
vitamin D	400 IU
vitamin E	200 IU
vitamin C	200 mg
folic acid	200 μg
thiamin (B_1)	25 mg
riboflavin (B_2)	25 mg
niacin	25 mg
vitamin B_6	25 mg
vitamin B_{12}	25 μg
biotin	25 μg
pantothenic acid	25 mg
calcium	200 mg
phosphorus	152 mg
iron	18 mg
magnesium	50 mg
copper	0.5 mg
zinc	15 mg
potassium	30 mg
choline	25 mg
inositol	25 mg
para-aminobenzoic acid	25 mg

| chromium | 7.5 μg |
| selenium | 12.5 μg |

Comments:

- This product provides greater than 100 percent of the U.S. RDA for vitamin E, vitamin C, niacin, B_{12}, biotin, and pantothenic acid.
- This product provides megadoses (ten times or more of the US RDA) for thiamin, riboflavin, B_6, and biotin.
- Accidental iron poisoning is a real possibility, especially with young children. *Keep all supplements out of their reach.*

SPAN-FF (iron supplement)

Manufacturer: Metro Med, Inc.
Dosage form: Capsules
Ingredients:

| elemental iron | 106 mg |

Comments:

- This product provides greater than 100 percent of the U.S. RDA.
- Accidental iron poisoning is a real possibility, especially with young children. *Keep all supplements stored out of their reach.*
- This supplement should not be used by people with peptic ulcer, regional enteritis, or ulcerative colitis.

Supplement Product Profiles

SPARTUS
(multivitamin/mineral supplement)

Manufacturer: Lederle Laboratories
Dosage form: Tablets
Ingredients:

vitamin A	5,000 IU
vitamin E	30 IU
vitamin C	300 mg
folic acid	400 μg
thiamin (B$_1$)	500 mg
riboflavin (B$_2$)	8.5 mg
niacin	100 mg
vitamin B$_6$	10 mg
vitamin B$_{12}$	30 μg
vitamin D	400 IU
biotin	45 μg
pantothenic acid	25 mg
iodine	150 μg
magnesium	100 mg
copper	2 mg
chromium	25 μg
molybdenum	25 μg
selenium	25 μg
manganese	5 mg
potassium	40 mg
chloride	36.3 mg
zinc	15 mg
calcium	162 mg
phosphorus	75 mg

Comments:
- This product provides greater than 100 percent of the U.S. RDA for vitamin C, thiamin, riboflavin,

niacin, B_6, B_{12}, and pantothenic acid.
- This supplement contains sucrose.

SPARTUS + IRON
(multivitamin/mineral supplement with iron)

Manufacturer: Lederle Laboratories
Dosage form: Tablets
Ingredients:
  Contains the same nutrients as SPARTUS, with the addition of 27 mg of iron.
Comments:
- This product provides greater than 100 percent of the U.S. RDA for vitamin C, thiamin, riboflavin, niacin, B_6, B_{12}, pantothenic acid, and iron.
- Accidental iron poisoning is a real possibility, especially with young children. *Keep all supplements out of their reach.*

STRESSGARD
(multivitamin/mineral supplement)

Manufacturer: Miles Laboratories, Inc.
Dosage form: Tablets
Ingredients:

vitamin A	5,000 IU
vitamin C	600 mg
thiamin (B_1)	15 mg
riboflavin (B_2)	10 mg
niacin	100 mg
vitamin D	400 IU

Supplement Product Profiles

vitamin E	30 IU
vitami B$_6$	5 mg
folic acid	400 µg
vitamin B$_{12}$	12 µg
pantothenic acid	20 mg
elemental iron	18 mg
zinc	15 mg
copper	2 mg

Comments:

- This product provides greater than 100 percent of the U.S. RDA for riboflavin, niacin, B$_6$, B$_{12}$, and pantothenic acid.
- This provides megadoses (ten or more times the U.S. RDA) for vitamin C and thiamin.
- Accidental iron poisoning is a real possibility, especially with young children. *Keep all supplements stored out of their reach.*

STRESSTABS 600 ADVANCED
(multivitamin supplement)

Manufacturer: Lederle Laboratories
Dosage form: Tablets
Ingredients:

vitamin E	30 IU
vitamin C	600 mg
folic acid	400 µg
thiamin (B$_1$)	15 mg
riboflavin (B$_2$)	10 mg
niacin	100 mg
vitamin B$_6$	5 mg
vitamin B$_{12}$	12 µg

| biotin | 45 µg |
| pantothenic acid | 20 mg |

Comments:

- This product provides greater than 100 percent of the U.S. RDA for riboflavin, niacin, B_6, B_{12}, and pantothenic acid.
- This product provides a megadose (ten or more times the U.S. RDA) for vitamin C and thiamin.

STRESSTABS 600 + IRON
(multivitamin supplement with iron)

Manufacturer: Lederle Laboratories
Dosage form: Tablets
Ingredients:

Contains the same ingredients as STRESSTABS 600 ADVANCED, with the addition of 27 mg of iron.

Comments:

- Provides greater than 100 percent of the US RDA for riboflavin, niacin, B_6, B_{12}, pantothenic acid and iron.
- Provides a megadose (ten or more times the US RDA) for vitamin C and thiamin.
- Accidental iron poisoning is a real possibility, especially with young children. *Keep all supplements stored out of their reach.*

STRESSTABS 600 + ZINC
(multivitamin/mineral supplement)

Manufacturer: Lederle Laboratories
Dosage form: Tablets

Supplement Product Profiles

Ingredients:
Contains the same ingredients as STRESSTABS 600 ADVANCED, with the addition of 3 mg of copper and 23.9 mg of zinc.

Comments:
- This product provides greater than 100 percent of the U.S. RDA for riboflavin, niacin, B_6, B_{12}, pantothenic acid, copper, and zinc.
- This product provides a megadose (ten or more times the U.S. RDA) for vitamin C and thiamin.

STUART FORMULA, THE
(multivitamin/mineral supplement)

Manufacturer: Stuart Pharmaceuticals
Dosage form: Tablets
Ingredients:

vitamin A	5,000 IU
vitamin D	400 IU
vitamin E	15 IU
vitamin C	60 mg
folic acid	400 µg
thiamin (B_1)	1.5 mg
riboflavin (B_2)	1.7 mg
niacin	20 mg
vitamin B_6	2 mg
vitamin B_{12}	6 µg
calcium	160 mg
phosphorus	125 mg
iodine	150 µg
elemental iron	18 mg
magnesium	100 mg

Comments:
- Accidental iron poisoning is a real possibility, especially with young children. *Keep all supplements stored out of their reach.*
- This supplement contains sugar.

STUART PRENATAL
(multivitamin/mineral supplement)

Manufacturer: Stuart Pharmaceuticals
Dosage form: Tablets
Ingredients:

vitamin A	8,000 IU
vitamin D	400 IU
vitamin E	30 IU
vitamin C	60 mg
folic acid	800 μg
thiamin (B_1)	1.7 mg
riboflavin (B_2)	2 mg
niacin	20 mg
vitamin B_6	4 mg
vitamin B_{12}	8 μg
calcium	200 mg
iodine	150 μg
elemental iron	60 mg
magnesium	100 mg
zinc	25 mg

Comments:
- This product provides 100 percent of the U.S. RDA for pregnant and breast-feeding women for vitamin A, vitamin D, vitamin E, vitamin C, folic acid, thiamin, riboflavin, niacin, B_{12}, and iodine.

Supplement Product Profiles

- This product provides greater than 100 percent of the U.S. RDA for B_6, iron, and zinc.
- This supplement contains FD&C Red No. 3, whose safety as a food colorant is in question.
- Accidental iron poisoning is a real possibility, especially with young children. *Keep all supplements stored out of their reach.*

STUARTINIC
(iron + multivitamin supplement)

Manufacturer: Stuart Pharmaceuticals
Dosage form: Tablets
Ingredients:

elemental iron	100 mg
vitamin C	500 mg
vitamin B_{12}	25 μg
thiamin (B_1)	6 mg
riboflavin (B_2)	6 mg
vitamin B_6	1 mg
niacin	20 mg
pantothenic acid	10 mg

Comments:
- This product provides greater than 100 percent of the U.S. RDA for iron, vitamin C, B_{12}, thiamin, and riboflavin.
- Accidental iron poisoning is a real possibility, especially with young children. *Keep all supplements stored out of their reach.*

Supplement Product Profiles

SUNKIST VITAMIN C (vitamin C supplement)

Manufacturer: CIBA Consumer Pharmaceuticals
Dosage form: Chewable tablets, caplets
Ingredients:

vitamin C	60 mg tablet
	250 mg tablet
	500 mg tablet
	500 mg caplet

Comments:
- 60 mg tablet provides 100 percent of the U.S. RDA.
- 250 mg tablet, 500 mg tablet, and 500 mg caplet provide greater than 100 percent of the U.S. RDA.
- Long-term use of high-dose chewable vitamin C tablets has been linked to erosion of dental enamel.

SUPLICAL (calcium supplement)

Manufacturer: Parke-Davis
Dosage form: Chewable tablets
Ingredients:

elemental calcium	600 mg

Comments: This product contains sugar, sorbitol, and hydrolyzed milk protein.

Supplement Product Profiles

SUPLICAL + D
(calcium supplement with vitamin D)

Manufacturer: Parke-Davis
Dosage form: Chewable tablets
Ingredients:

elemental calcium	600 mg
vitamin D	125 IU

Comments: This product contains sugar, sorbitol, and hydrolyzed milk protein.

SURBEX (multivitamin supplement)

Manufacturer: Abbott Laboratories
Dosage form: Tablets
Ingredients:

niacin	30 mg
pantothenic acid	10 mg
thiamin (B_1)	6 mg
riboflavin (B_2)	6 mg
vitamin B_6	2.5 mg
vitamin B_{12}	5 μg

Comments: This product provides greater than 100 percent of the U.S. RDA for niacin, thiamin, riboflavin, and B_6.

SURBEX WITH C
(multivitamin supplement)

Manufacturer: Abbott Laboratories
Dosage form: Tablets

Ingredients:

Contains the same ingredients as SURBEX, with the addition of 250 mg of vitamin C.

Comments: This product provides greater than 100 percent of the U.S. RDA for niacin, thiamin, riboflavin, B_6, and vitamin C.

SURBEX-T (multivitamin supplement)

Manufacturer: Abbott Laboratories
Dosage form: Tablets
Ingredients:

vitamin C	500 mg
niacin	100 mg
pantothenic acid	20 mg
thiamin (B_1)	15 mg
riboflavin (B_2)	10 mg
vitamin B_6	5 mg
vitamin B_{12}	10 μg

Comments:

● This product provides greater than 100 percent of the U.S. RDA for vitamin C, niacin, pantothenic acid, riboflavin, B_6, and B_{12}.

● This product provides a megadose (ten or more times the U.S. RDA) for thiamin.

SURBEX-750 WITH IRON (multivitamin supplement plus iron)

Manufacturer: Abbott Laboratories
Dosage form: Tablets

Supplement Product Profiles

Ingredients:

vitamin C	750 mg
niacin	100 mg
vitamin B_6	25 mg
pantothenic acid	20 mg
thiamin (B_1)	15 mg
riboflavin (B_2)	15 mg
vitamin B_{12}	12 μg
folic acid	400 μg
vitamin E	30 IU
elemental iron	27 mg

Comments:

- This product provides greater than 100 percent of the U.S. RDA for niacin, pantothenic acid, riboflavin, B_{12}, and iron.
- This product provides a megadose (ten or more times the U.S. RDA) for vitamin C, B_6, and thiamin.
- Accidental iron poisoning is a real possibility, especially with young children. *Keep all supplements stored out of their reach.*

SURBEX-750 WITH ZINC
(multivitamin supplement plus zinc)

Manufacturer: Abbott Laboratories
Dosage form: Tablets
Ingredients:

vitamin C	750 mg
niacin	100 mg
vitamin B_6	20 mg
pantothenic acid	20 mg
thiamin (B_1)	15 mg
riboflavin (B_2)	15 mg

vitamin B_{12}	12 µg
folic acid	400 µg
vitamin E	30 IU
zinc	22.5 mg

Comments:

- This product provides greater than 100 percent of the U.S RDA for riboflavin, niacin, B_{12}, pantothenic acid, and zinc.
- This product provides a megadose (ten or more times the U.S. RDA) for vitamin C, thiamin, and B_6.

SUSTAINED RELEASE VITA-C 500
(vitamin C supplement)

Manufacturer: Shaklee Corporation
Dosage form: Tablets
Ingredients:

vitamin C	500 mg

Comments:

- This product provides greater than 100 percent of the U.S. RDA vitamin C.
- This product is Kosher certified.

THERA-COMBEX H-P
(multivitamin supplement)

Manufacturer: Parke-Davis
Dosage form: Capsules
Ingredients:

vitamin C	500 mg
thiamin (B_1)	25 mg
riboflavin (B_2)	15 mg

Supplement Product Profiles

vitamin B_6	10 mg
vitamin B_{12}	5 μg
niacin	100 mg
pantothenic acid	20 mg

Comments:
- This product provides greater than the U.S. RDA for vitamin C, riboflavin, B_6, niacin, and pantothenic acid.
- This product provides a megadose (ten or more times the U.S. RDA) for thiamin.

THERAGRAM LIQUID
(multivitamin supplement)

Manufacturer: E.R. Squibb & Sons, Inc.
Dosage form: Liquid
Ingredients:

vitamin A	10,000 IU
vitamin D	400 IU
vitamin C	200 mg
thiamin (B_1)	10 mg
riboflavin (B_2)	10 mg
niacin	100 mg
vitamin B_6	4.1 mg
vitamin B_{12}	5 μg
pantothenic acid	21.4 mg

Comments: This product provides greater than the U.S. RDA for vitamin A, vitamin C, thiamin, riboflavin, niacin, B_6, and pantothenic acid.

THERAGRAM STRESS FORMULA
(multivitamin supplement with iron)

Manufacturer: E.R. Squibb & Sons, Inc.
Dosage form: Tablets
Ingredients:

vitamin E	30 IU
vitamin C	600 mg
folic acid	400 µg
thiamin (B_1)	15 mg
riboflavin (B_2)	15 mg
niacin	100 mg
vitamin B_6	25 mg
vitamin B_{12}	12 µg
biotin	45 µg
pantothenic acid	20 mg
iron	27 mg

Comments:
- This product provides greater than the U.S. RDA for riboflavin, niacin, B_{12}, pantothenic acid, and iron.
- This product provides megadoses (ten or more times the U.S. RDA) for vitamin C, thiamin, and B_6.
- Accidental iron poisoning is a real possibility, especially with young children. *Keep all supplements stored out of their reach.*

THERAGRAM TABLETS ADVANCED FORMULA (multivitamin supplement)

Manufacturer: E.R. Squibb & Sons, Inc.
Dosage form: Tablets

Supplement Product Profiles

Ingredients:

vitamin A	5,500 IU
vitamin C	120 mg
thiamin (B_1)	3 mg
riboflavin (B_2)	3.4 mg
niacin	30 mg
vitamin B_6	3 mg
vitamin B_{12}	9 µg
vitamin D	400 IU
vitamin E	30 IU
pantothenic acid	10 mg
folic acid	400 µg
biotin	15 µg

Comments: This product provides greater than the U.S. RDA for vitamin A, vitamin C, thiamin, riboflavin, niacin, B_6, and B_{12}.

THERAGRAM-M ADVANCED FORMULA
(multivitamin/mineral supplement)

Manufacturer: E.R. Squibb & Sons, Inc.
Dosage form: Tablets
Ingredients:

vitamin A	5,500 IU
vitamin C	120 mg
thiamin (B_1)	3 mg
riboflavin (B_2)	3.4 mg
niacin	30 mg
vitamin B_6	3 mg
vitamin B_{12}	9 µg

vitamin D	400 IU
vitamin E	30 IU
pantothenic acid	10 mg
folic acid	400 µg
biotin	15 µg
calcium	40 mg
iodine	150 µg
iron	27 mg
magnesium	100 mg
copper	2 mg
zinc	15 mg
manganese	5 mg
chromium	15 µg
selenium	10 µg
molybdenum	15 µg
phosphorus	31 mg
potassium	7.5 mg
chloride	7.5 mg

Comments:

- This product provides greater than 100 percent of the U.S. RDA for vitamin A, vitamin C, thiamin, riboflavin, niacin, B_6, B_{12}, and iron.
- Accidental iron poisoning is a real possibility, especially with young children. *Keep all supplements stored out of their reach.*

TRI-VI-SOL (multivitamin supplement)

Manufacturer: Mead Johnson Nutritional Division
Dosage form: Liquid

Supplement Product Profiles

Ingredients:

vitamin A	1,500 IU
vitamin D	400 IU
vitamin C	35 mg

Comments: This product provides 100 percent of the U.S. RDA for infants for each nutrient.

TRI-VI-SOL WITH IRON
(multivitamin supplement with iron)

Manufacturer: Mead Johnson Nutritional Division
Dosage form: Liquid
Ingredients:
Contains the same ingredients as TRI-VI-SOL, with the addition of 10 mg of iron.
Comments: Accidental iron poisoning is a real possibility, especially with young children. *Keep all supplements stored out of their reach.*

TROPH-IRON B
(vitamin supplement with iron)

Manufacturer: SmithKline Consumer Products
Dosage form: Liquid
Ingredients:

thiamin (B_1)	10 mg
vitamin B_{12}	25 µg
iron	20 mg

Comments:
- This product provides greater than 100 percent of the U.S. RDA for each nutrient.
- This supplement contains sugar.

- This product contains FD&C Red No. 40, whose safety as a food colorant is still in question.
- Accidental iron poisoning is a real possibility, especially with young children. *Keep all supplements stored out of their reach.*
- Iron interferes with the absorption of oral tetracycline antibiotics and may reduce the effectiveness of the drug.
- This supplement may cause nausea, constipation, or diarrhea.
- Contact your pharmacist or physician for further information.

TROPHITE B (vitamin supplement)

Manufacturer: SmithKline Consumer Products
Dosage form: Liquid, tablets
Ingredients:

thiamin (B_1)	10 mg
vitamin B_{12}	25 µg

Comments: This product provides greater than 100 percent of the U.S. RDA for both vitamins.

UNICAP (multivitamin supplement)

Manufacturer: The Upjohn Company
Dosage form: Tablets, capsules
Ingredients:

vitamin A	5,000 IU
vitamin D	400 IU
vitamin E	15 IU
vitamin C	60 mg

Supplement Product Profiles

folic acid	400 μg
thiamin (B$_1$)	1.5 mg
riboflavin (B$_2$)	1.7 mg
niacin	20 mg
vitamin B$_6$	2 mg
vitamin B$_{12}$	6 μg

Comments:

- This product provides 100 percent of the U.S. RDA for each nutrient except vitamin E, for which less is provided.
- This supplement is sugar and sodium free.

UNICAP JR (multivitamin supplement)

Manufacturer: The Upjohn Company
Dosage form: Chewable tablets
Ingredients:
Contains the same ingredients as UNICAP.
Comments:

- This product provides 100 percent of the U.S. RDA for each nutrient except vitamin E, for which less is provided.
- This supplement contains sugar and mannitol.

UNICAP M
(multivitamin/mineral supplement)

Manufacturer: The Upjohn Company
Dosage form: Tablets
Ingredients:

vitamin A	5,000 IU
vitamin D	400 IU

vitamin E	30 IU
vitamin C	60 mg
folic acid	400 μg
thiamin (B_1)	1.5 mg
riboflavin (B_2)	1.7 mg
niacin	20 mg
vitamin B_6	2 mg
vitamin B_{12}	6 μg
pantothenic acid	10 mg
iodine	150 μg
iron	18 mg
copper	2 mg
zinc	15 mg
calcium	60 mg
phosphorus	45 mg
manganese	1 mg
potassium	5 mg

Comments:
- This product provides 100 percent or less of the U.S. RDA for each nutrient.
- This supplement is sugar and sodium free.

UNICAP PLUS IRON
(multivitamin supplement with iron)

Manufacturer: The Upjohn Company
Dosage form: Tablets
Ingredients:
Contains the same vitamins in the same amounts as UNICAP M with only one mineral, iron.
Comments:
- This product provides 100 percent of the U.S. RDA for each nutrient.

Supplement Product Profiles

- This supplement contains sugar.
- Accidental iron poisoning is a real possibility, especially with young children. *Keep all supplements stored out of their reach.*

UNICAP SENIOR
(multivitamin/mineral supplement)

Manufacturer: The Upjohn Company
Dosage form: Tablets
Ingredients:

vitamin A	5,000 IU
vitamin D	200 IU
vitamin E	15 IU
vitamin C	60 mg
folic acid	400 µg
thiamin (B_1)	1.2 mg
riboflavin (B_2)	1.4 mg
niacin	16 mg
vitamin B_6	2.2 mg
vitamin B_{12}	3 µg
pantothenic acid	10 mg
iodine	150 µg
iron	10 mg
copper	2 mg
zinc	15 mg
calcium	100 mg
phosphorus	77 mg
magnesium	30 mg
manganese	1 mg
potassium	5 mg

Comments:
- This supplement is sugar and sodium free.
- Accidental iron poisoning is a real possibility, especially with young children. *Keep all supplements stored out of their reach.*

UNICAP T
(multivitamin/mineral supplement)

Manufacturer: The Upjohn Company
Dosage form: Tablets
Ingredients:

vitamin A	5,000 IU
vitamin D	400 IU
vitamin E	30 IU
vitamin C	500 mg
folic acid	400 µg
thiamin (B_1)	10 mg
riboflavin (B_2)	10 mg
niacin	100 mg
vitamin B_6	6 mg
vitamin B_{12}	18 µg
pantothenic acid	25 mg
iodine	150 µg
iron	18 mg
copper	2 mg
zinc	15 mg
manganese	1 mg
potassium	5 mg
selenium	10 µg

Supplement Product Profiles

Comments:
- This product provides greater than 100 percent of the U.S. RDA for vitamin C, thiamin, riboflavin, niacin, B_6, B_{12}, and pantothenic acid.
- This supplement is sugar and sodium free.

VI-PENTA INFANT DROPS
(multivitamin supplement)

Manufacturer: Roche Laboratories
Dosage form: Liquid
Ingredients:

vitamin A	5,000 IU
vitamin D	400 IU
vitamin C	50 mg
vitamin E	2 IU

Comments:
- This product provides greater than 100 percent of the U.S. RDA for infants under 1 year for vitamin A and vitamin C.
- It provides greater than 100 percent of the U.S. RDA for children under age 4 for vitamin A and vitamin C.

VI-PENTA MULTIVITAMIN DROPS
(multivitamin supplement)

Manufacturer: Roche Laboratories
Dosage form: Liquid
Ingredients:

vitamin A	5,000 IU
vitamin D	400 IU

vitamin C	50 mg
thiamin (B$_1$)	I mg
riboflavin (B$_2$)	I mg
vitamin B$_6$	I mg
vitamin E	2 IU
biotin	30 μg
niacin	10 mg
pantothenic acid	10 mg

Comments: This product provides greater than 100 percent of the U.S. RDA for infants and children under the age of 4 for vitamin A, vitamin C, thiamin, riboflavin, niacin, and pantothenic acid.

VITA-LEA (multivitamin/mineral supplement)

Manufacturer: Shaklee Corporation
Dosage form: Tablets
Ingredients:

vitamin A	2,500 IU
vitamin D	200 IU
vitamin E	15 IU
vitamin C	45 mg
folic acid	200 μg
thiamin (B$_1$)	I mg
riboflavin (B$_2$)	I.2 mg
niacin	10 mg
vitamin B$_6$	2 mg
vitamin B$_{12}$	4.5 μg
biotin	0.15 mg
pantothenic acid	5 mg
calcium	300 mg
phosphorus	225 mg

Supplement Product Profiles

iodine	75 μg
iron	9 mg
magnesium	100 mg
copper	1 mg
zinc	15 mg

Comments:

- Accidental iron poisoning is real possibility, especially with young children. *Keep all supplements stored out of their reach.*
- This product is Kosher certified.

VITAMIN C WITH ROSE HIPS
(vitamin C supplement)

Manufacturer: Nature Made Nutritional Products
Dosage form: Tablets, chewable tablets
Ingredients:
    Tablets:
        vitamin C   250 mg;   750 mg;
                        1,000 mg; 1,500 mg
    Chewable tablets:
        vitamin C   300 mg; 500 mg

Comments:

- 250 mg tablets, and 300 mg and 500 mg chewable tablets provide greater than 100 percent of the U.S. RDA for vitamin C.
- 750 mg, 1,000 mg, and 1,500 mg tablets provide a megadose (ten or more times the U.S. RDA) for vitamin C.
- Long-term use of high-dose chewable vitamin C tablets has been associated with dental erosion.

Supplement Product Profiles

VITAMIN E (vitamin E supplement)

Manufacturer: Nature Made Nutritional Products
Dosage form: Capsules
Ingredients:

vitamin E	200 IU; 400 IU; 600 IU; 1,000 IU

Comments:
- 200 IU capsules provide greater than 100 percent of the U.S. RDA.
- 400 IU, 600 IU, and 1,000 IU provide a megadose (ten or more times the U.S. RDA).

WITHIN
(multivitamin/mineral supplement)

Manufacturer: Miles Laboratories, Inc.
Dosage form: Tablets
Ingredients:

vitamin A	5,000 IU
vitamin C	60 mg
thiamin (B_1)	1.5 mg
riboflavin (B_2)	1.7 mg
niacin	20 mg
vitamin D	400 IU
vitamin E	30 IU
vitamin B_6	2 mg
folic acid	400 μg
vitamin B_{12}	6 μg
pantothenic acid	10 mg
elemental iron	27 mg
elemental calcium	300 mg

Supplement Product Profiles

Comments:
- This product provides greater than 100 percent of the U.S. RDA for iron.
- Accidental iron poisoning is a real possibility, especially with young children. *Keep all supplements stored out of their reach.*

Z-BEC
(multivitamin supplement with zinc)

Manufacturer: A.H. Robins Company, Inc.
Dosage form: Tablets
Ingredients:

vitamin E	45 IU
vitamin C	600 mg
thiamin (B_1)	15 mg
riboflavin (B_2)	10.2 mg
niacin	100 mg
vitamin B_6	10 mg
vitamin B_{12}	6 μg
pantothenic acid	25 mg
zinc	22.5 mg

Comments:
- This product provides greater than 100 percent of the U.S. RDA for vitamin E, riboflavin, niacin, B6, pantothenic acid, and zinc.
- This product provides a megadose (ten or more times the U.S. RDA) for vitamin C and thiamin.

Index

Index

Index

Index

Index